SACRED SELF,
SACRED RELATIONSHIPS

Sacred Self, Sacred Relationships

Healing the World for Seven Generations

BLACKWOLF JONES and GINA JONES

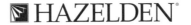

Hazelden
Center City, Minnesota 55012-0176

1-800-328-0094
1-651-213-4590 (Fax)
www.hazelden.org

ISBN: 1-56838-789-X

06 05 04 03 02 6 5 4 3 2 1

Cover design by Lightbourne
Interior design and typesetting by Terri Kinne

Our love and hope go out to the children
of the next seven generations.

Contents

Acknowledgments

We would like to thank the people who have passed their understandings on to us throughout the years. From elders to professors to friends and family, we respectfully honor their wisdom.

We would also like to thank our editor, Richard Solly, for his patience, foresight, and eye for detail. As our first reader and critic, we honor his contributions.

We extend a big thank-you to our children for their patience and understanding as this book was being written and rewritten.

Finally, we would like to thank our Creator.

Introduction

A pebble drops into a still lake, reverberates farther and farther out from here and now, and touches the shores of distant times and places. Concentric circles ripple—vibrate—with just one touch.

This book is about these circles: where and how they start, where and how they go. Just as one moment of health promotes greater health, one pinpoint of hurt may also reach out to hurt others. Circles of help or hurt are created, always. It is one or the other.

To become skillful with relationships with self and others, a circular vision is required. Unless we begin to see around us, within us, and beyond us, we unwittingly continue cycles of abuse, whether as victims or perpetrators. We are either part of the circle of abuse, or we are part of the circle of healing. We cannot avoid the circle. We cannot avoid the ripples.

Circular vision is not something new. It is old. The circle, a universal archetype, has been a focal point for spiritual traditions for thousands of years. The circle symbolizes birth and rebirth, cycles, and completeness. Even more, it teaches us how to see and live life. Circular vision is inclusive, rather than exclusive, just as there are no limits to the circle's ripples. Insight complements foresight and hindsight. But there is more. Beyond looking ahead, behind, and within us, circular vision requires us to look around and out. Relationships—healthy relationships, *sacred* relationships—require this type of vision. When we see life with circular vision, things change.

Imagine a circle of thirty sixth-grade students, all thinking and feeling beyond their own personal circumstances. It seems nearly impossible. Thirty kids at the same time? Thirty preadolescents? Even one student doing so, hormones raging, would be a feat in our self-centered, self-indulgent, dysfunctional, advertising, consuming world.

Now imagine these children not only thinking and feeling beyond self, but actually thinking and feeling into the next generation—imagining life years from now, mentally experiencing the consequences of their actions and inactions. Then on to the next generation, and the next, and further out until finally all thirty children are thinking and feeling into the seventh generation—a time when their bodies will no longer exist as they are now here on this earth, a time beyond their personal gain. Now, imagine them caring. Truly. Can this happen? Can thirty preadolescents possess the ability and the wisdom to *collectively* reach beyond their lives in such a profound way?

Yes. We have seen it happen. We have witnessed it. They saw with circular vision.

Indigenous people of this land understood this type of vision. All major Iroquoian decisions, for example, were based upon the principle of the seventh generation. As a guiding principle, the Iroquois relied on the circle.

When a decision was needed, the council came together in a talking circle, and the sacred eagle feather was passed around. The person who held the feather gained the total attention and respect of the group. No interruptions. No time constraints. No one person held more power than another. Equality was honored. The talking circle, with circular vision that reached back into the past and forward into the future, patiently came to a consensus, to one mind. Simply stated, if an action would help the seventh generation to come, then the decision was supported by the council. If a decision would hurt the seventh generation, then it would be avoided.

Passing this profound teaching from Iroquoian ancestors on to our students and clients here in the United States, and now around the world, has become perhaps the most uplifting experience in our careers. After seeing others think and feel with circular vision, we have often asked them, "What would change if the world made all decisions based on the principle of the seventh generation?"

Everything would change!

Adults' and children's attitudes, commitment, and awareness unfold before our very eyes. Sincerity and an understanding of relationships emerge. Long-lasting respect and honor for self and others continue to echo, even now, years later. With the seeds planted, we are certain that a difference *is* being made—not only for our students' and clients' personal happiness, but also in the lives of the unborn. It is there. We know.

Sacred Self, Sacred Relationships invites you to look into self and out to the seventh generation, asking you to see, if for the first time, with circular vision. The world will undoubtedly look very different; as if you are seeing three-dimensional objects hidden in optical illusions for the first time, you may come away with a feeling of great discovery.

What you do today does and will affect not only your life, but also the generations to come. What you choose and what you say, every moment, is a gift. You have chosen to pick up this book. Do you feel the circles rippling out? What circles are you beginning? Remember, it begins with you, with your happiness.

There are many paths to walk, many choices to be made, many options to consider. Too often, we only follow what we already know, what we are familiar and comfortable with. Too often, we find ourselves in a rut, not on a journey. Come and discover healthy options for yourself, even if, in doing so, you must let go of what you know.

Life has always emerged from the unknown, the unfamiliar, the darkness. Each child to be born is an unknown spirit. Each sprout from the spring ground emerges from darkness and mystery. Each breath we accept goes back to fulfill that which we do not know. Each breath does not guarantee the next. Our very existence—our very beings—are mysteries; the ripples we set in motion will arrive on distant shores at distant times.

As you read through this book you will notice the use of the pronoun "we", meant to simplify the reading. To continuously separate one author's experience from the other would divide the spirit of this book. Nonetheless, from time to time, it is necessary to identify one author. These distinctions of unique life experiences complement true unity of spirit.

This book embraces and honors the mystery of who you are, who we all are, and the relationships that we develop. Relationships imply fluidity and mystery. Otherwise, life would be but a script. Accept the mystery and witness how your life unfolds. This book will empower and celebrate you and your potential while training your spiritual eyes to see beyond this moment, thereby promoting healthy relationships with all of life.

We invite you to come along and discover the sacred in all your relationships—the mysteries, the reverberations, the circles of seven generations and beyond.

PART ONE

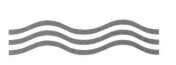

BUILDING
AWARENESS
OF SELF

Chapter One

A Time to Trust

Your circle begins with awareness, and your awareness is stirred up upon awakening. How did you wake up today? To an alarm clock? To the birds singing outside your window? To the noise in the next room? When and how did your awareness begin? Did you miss the sunrise? Did you catch the sunrise? Did you even think about the sunrise?

Sadly, in a compulsive attempt to capture that which is outside self, many miss the moment that can occur only within personal beginnings. When will you attend to your own sunrise and becoming?

Necessary changes must take place as you prepare for your personal transformation. Awareness first within—an internal sunrise—must occur before you are capable of truly appreciating the movement outside yourself. Look and listen within before you look and listen outside yourself. Wake up and marvel at who you are.

Mindfulness—thinking about your thinking, doing, and being—becomes a catalyst and will assist you in the necessary work to be done. New awareness, or the *mind of the beginner,* is the first necessary stepping-stone to empowerment.

Awakening (unlike awareness, which is an eternal aspect of your being) is the prerequisite to change. This awakening is the pebble in the water to your own healing and transformation.

Without this, there is no contact. Without contact, there are no ripples to effectively and positively change your experience. Awakening becomes the center of your circle.

Time no longer matters when you deliberately journey to the center of your own existence. Here, in the silence of being, listening, attending, and witnessing, you see your life from afar. Here, in the center of your existence, you recognize mysteries that await spiritual awareness. So begin in your silence and listen to the story of ancient times, the songs of ancestors, the rhythm of Mother Earth. Reside in your own heart, in your own silence, in your own pain and joy. Come to your personal healing.

Your relationship with all that is outside you first depends on your relationship with yourself.

There will never be a better time than now to do what you know you need to do. What is it? You know! Have you listened? Do you trust? Now is the beginning. Welcome to coming home to yourself. Trust is truly the fundamental foundation to future growth—yours and others'. Once you experience the power behind such a simple yet sometimes difficult act, you will forever be a follower of this basic tenet of trust.

You know the word *trust*. But do you really know it personally? It is typical to trust others rather than yourself; to see stillness outside but not within; to applaud difficult transformation yet stubbornly refuse to change; to celebrate events outside yourself rather than those within. Too often, we are spectators of others' lives. We trust celebrities, athletes, heroes, and leaders as evidence of all that is possible. As spectators, however, we do not experience life; we don't trust *our* life within. Stillness, transcendence, transformation, and celebration are rarely perceived and experienced as events that occur within. Come to see that trust is the finest gift you must first give yourself.

It is easy to avoid change. The most decisive action is inaction, for it covertly leads us down paths of regret. The irony is that inaction is often disguised as being busy, while true transformation and purpose require the prerequisite of stillness and trust. We invite you to become an eager explorer willing to listen to the voice within. Here, your decisions will be guided, your experiences opened to views of sacred intention. Joseph Campbell, a renowned spiritual historian, refers to it as the invisible hand guiding your path, opening doors, making opportunities.

However, *you* must take the first step.

Even the whirlwind of life has a silent center, like the eye of a storm. Too often, we do not give ourselves this gift of presence. The eternal invitation awaits, however, for us all. And the gifts of this gift are life changing. The transformation of self-awareness into knowing occurs within the cocoon of trust and opens as wings of celebration. Trust leads to stillness, to transformation, to celebration. *Shh.* Listen. It all begins with trust.

Like an infant maneuvering within a new world, all personal transformation begins with trust. Trust implies confident reliance upon the future. Trust is expecting the best from life, expecting the best from yourself. Trust is feeling the unseen hand guide your future. It is all one and the same.

Trust.

Although we walk within it and sleep within it, too often we talk and think and do *without* it. We have become distracted *from* and have become blind and deaf *to* the joy of personal and universal trust, thereby diminishing potential transformation and celebration. Any celebrated feat or adventure—be it ballooning around the world, creating a piece of art, or surviving horrendous difficulties—began with trust.

Offer your internal voice and ear as an avenue of beginning. With your spiritual eye, consider unfathomed possibilities.

Trust! Trust in yourself, in the world, in the eternal. Learn to appreciate the mind of the beginner. Indeed, celebrate new beginnings, exciting possibilities, and the journey of your spiritual innocence. Reach beyond and remember within; honor stillness and movement. Dig in! Trust the journey. Trust *your* journey. Surrender to a power greater than you, for the gifts are tremendous.

Authentic pride and true integrity are begotten of trust. Trust your mistakes, for they carry messages of direction. A sense of knowing epitomizes a developed self-awareness. Emerge from the eternal cocoon that you know exists for yourself. Pause. Listen. Trust. Change. Celebrate. Hear and be heard. Certainty in today's world is rare, but real. Right now, recognize there is a time to be still. When you find yourself on a path divided, be still and listen. It is a crucial moment. Trust. *Without* it, you may distract yourself from exciting possibilities. *Within* it, you can listen and discover your destiny. Trust your wings and celebrate the journey. There will never be a better time to fly and maybe never another opportunity.

In essence, Socrates invited us to *know* ourselves. Do you know yourself? Freud urged us to *be* ourselves. Are you becoming yourself? Jesus, along with many other spiritual leaders, asks us to *give* ourselves. Do you give of yourself? Do you hear the voices of the future in these words of our beloved spiritual leaders? Do you hear the "we-ness" of the seventh generation? Do you trust yourself, others, and the universe enough to make today's decisions ensure the future welfare of the next seven generations—your children, their children, their children, their children, their children, their children, and their children? These three tenets—to know yourself, to be yourself, and to give yourself—are all born of trust.

Escort yourself right now to a moment of silence, to your

eternal being. Please pause and listen. Trust and connect to the future.

Know Self

The eyes of the children are watching. Who we are, how we feel about ourselves, what we personally do or do not, matters. Our personal, isolated lives reverberate throughout the universe. Each individual affects the children of today, the children of tomorrow—indeed, the child within us.

Think of what you have chosen to do today. What was it? Did you make a meal, earn a living, offer a smile, lend a hand? Think now on how your decisions and attitudes, just for today, mattered to those who share your space. Today, someone gave up a parking space to an elder. Today, someone brought laughter. Today, someone made a healthy soup. Today, someone volunteered as a plasma donor at the Red Cross. Think now on how these same choices affected your experience of the world today and will influence the world tomorrow. Tomorrow, you could be the recipient.

You may find it helpful to look back at yourself with a child's wide-eyed awareness. If you need a reason to improve your relationship with yourself, here is a noble one: do it for the children to come. If your body and emotions, through disease or stress and tension, have already given you signals to read further, may this consideration of future generations give you even more inner strength and foresight as you begin the inward exploration that each of us inevitably takes, even if it begins and ends on our deathbeds.

But your personal self-discovery need not wait until the moment of your ultimate transformation. Although we undeniably realize that the most profound transformation will take place at the mystery of our death, transformation can begin here and now, for our very existence is a mystery that many of us have taken for granted. Why were you selected to exist here and now among an infinite number of other options?

Do you remember the moments, perhaps as a child or adolescent, when you asked philosophical questions? *Why am I here? Who am I? What is life? When did I begin? Will I end?* Celebrate the philosopher's mind that embraces the truth: *I am alive! I am part of something so great, so awesome, so big!*

Face tomorrow with the hopes and dreams of a child. Grab the moment and open the door to what may yet come. Is there a new job on the horizon? A new partner? A new family? A new home? A new journey? A new lifestyle? A new you? Take the steps necessary in order to grow. Know this will be difficult. Do not allow fears and discomfort to influence your decision to change. We would guess that astronauts' heart monitors reveal quickened heartbeats upon takeoff. To be alive is to be afraid sometimes. To be alive is to be uncomfortable sometimes, too.

Be willing to let go of unhealthy relationships or self-defeating tendencies. Be prepared to replace them with healthy patterns. Look forward to learning it all over again. Become a lifelong student of life. Refuse to become so set in your ways, as you age, that you can no longer be wrong. Be mistaken! It's okay. Realize you will mess up. Make mistakes and celebrate them, for you are not a mistake. Mistakes are teachers. Become familiar with the unfamiliar. Become more fully you in the process of journeying new uncharted lands. It is time for new beginnings. Introduce yourself to the unknown parts of yourself, not just with fear, but also with courage and delight.

With the mind of the beginner, with the fearless questioning of the child, with the intuitive wisdom gained from the journey from one world to the next, from the silence we all ultimately leave and return to, consider and dive into your own mystery. At the very least, you may unlock shackles that now chain you to a habitual pattern of powerlessness. At the very most, you may even touch the outer fringes of the spirit world, as we will all someday make this final journey.

In this book, we will lead you through a series of exercises and discussions that, we hope, will enable you to see yourself with new eyes. Engage each exercise with both truth and time, and you will feel as though you have been offered a new pair of glasses, one with the perfect prescription for you. Each exercise will be a great source of vision and empowerment, offering a genuine opportunity for internal growth and reawakening.

We will begin with you. How do you feel about yourself? Rate yourself on a scale from one to ten, one being terrible, ten being terrific. Where are you at this moment? Where were you yesterday? Where are you in general? Keep this estimation in mind, for we will return to it later in Part One.

Exercise

For our first exercise, please stand with your hands placed at the level of how tall you *feel* inside your body. Please, do this now. Stand up. Do not think about it. Just place your hands at the level you feel you are inside.

Where did your hands end up? At your shoulders? Your waist? Your hips? Your knees? Your ankles? Where your hands end up is an outward expression of your feelings of self-worth.

If your hands were level with the crown of your head, you find yourself among the fortunate few. If, like most readers, you're not so fortunate, your spirit needs to be restored. The distance between where you placed your hands and the top of your head represents a vacancy that your spirit and feelings of self-sufficiency once occupied. This vacancy, or void, in spirit-presence fills itself with fears and feelings of inferiority.

Low self-esteem may be due to family stress. Often, children do not receive the attention, affection, recognition and approval, encouragement, and security that are needed for them to develop self-worth and a positive sense of self. This often leads to a negative self-image, self-degradation, and self-destructive behavior patterns. Together, we will work to replace these negative self-images with positive truths, extinguishing your fears while rejuvenating your spirit.

How did this erosion of self-esteem take place? You were born a global ball of spiritual fire. You lived totally in the present, knew nothing of past or future focus, and had no fears. Well, then, what happened between then and now to create your present condition?

You were socialized in an abusive society. That's what happened. If you trip on this statement and don't believe you have been raised in an abusive society, we invite you to watch your local and national news on TV tonight, then reconsider whether violence and abuse isn't and hasn't been woven into the fabric of society. How could this permeating influence not have affected you?

Although abuse has been present in some form since the dawn of time, this system virtually came to America about five hundred years ago, as the internal cargo of European immigrants. These people, entrenched in their feudal system ideology, brought it with them as the only lifestyle they knew. They were fleeing a very oppressive, controlling, and persecuting European existence in hopes of becoming free, independent, and autonomous. However, they brought with them a deluded form of the abusive systems that they, in fact, were trying to escape. A male-dominant power and control hierarchy soon developed, and their children were born into a society based on judgment and domination over others, especially minorities. The society that sprang up mimicked the feudal system with slavery, child labor, and the unbridled exploitation of life, land, and resources. The commonly used term *landlord* comes directly from the aristocratic, have-and-have-not feudal system.

In the past, kings and queens, closely supported by the church and the enforcement of the military, held the power. The game of chess reflects this hierarchical system. Today's kings and queens are some CEOs and corporations that dominate and operate with little or no concern for the seventh generation. They are concerned with immediate gratification, power, control, and gain. It is all about profit and exploitation of resources, including people. The system has been modified over the centuries, but the pawns are still the people.

What does this have to do with you? Everything. If you were born and raised in America, you were socialized by this system. This system (not to be confused with the loving and heroic efforts of individuals, families, and groups) was never designed to add value. The system was designed to devalue. As this system passed from one generation to the next, the devaluation rules of socialization were also passed on. This abusive system flourishes today, and prisons cannot be built fast enough to contain the aftermath of spiritual decay. This unquestioned domination continues to devastate our population. Gangs are an outgrowth of a society that has left children feeling helpless, hopeless, disempowered, and forgotten. Not coincidentally, gangs are not as prevalent in affluent neighborhoods as they are in poverty-stricken neighborhoods. However, no matter where you find yourself in our society, or in the world, you are affected.

You, then, have been socialized by the remnants of the feudal-abuse system, and your value has been diminished by virtue of that system's designs. Your parents and grandparents were victims of that system, as well.

Remember, you were born a full and complete global ball of spiritual fire. You were valued for your uniqueness rather than what you did or did not do. You only knew to be yourself. You didn't degrade or devalue yourself, and you were content with just getting your basic needs met. However, as you matured, your parents and others expected things of you. An unwritten rule-book dictated what you could and could not do, when, and where. You were measured as good or bad, competent or incompetent, smart or slow, depending on performance. The work ethic, which places value on you for *what* you do, took its toll. No longer were you valued for self. You were criticized and praised for actions.

All children want to please their parents and significant others in order to get the needed attention, affection, recognition, and approval that validates them and creates a sense of being loved and accepted. When you performed an action or a behavior of which your parents didn't approve, you took that part of yourself they found unacceptable and placed it in an invisible backpack, so to speak, that you keep strapped to your being. Maybe you were criticized for being too wiggly, and you redirected that action and energy into your bag. Maybe you spilled your milk, soiled your diaper, were too noisy, didn't eat all your food. Bit by bit, piece by piece, self-degradation filled your backpack. Perhaps your brothers and sisters also fought for dominance and often devalued you. Then your preschool and elementary school experience took its toll.

Children can be vicious, and they may have told you your nose or hair looked funny. Mimicking judgmental attitudes of parents and society, they continued the cycle of abuse. Perhaps you began to unravel under these assaults. In middle school and high school you became categorized into groups representative of performance status and competence: gifted and talented, learning disordered, athletic, antisocial, emotionally disturbed, and so on. You were sliced and diced socially, psychologically, and emotionally, all of which affected you spiritually. This qualifying hierarchical structure continued to dominate. More and more of who you really were went in the backpack as an effort to please and be accepted, and less and less of your self-esteem survived. Some teachers may have added their innuendoes. Report cards may have spoken of your inadequacies.

You went off to college and experienced more of the same. Then came your first real job. Bosses, corporations, and the military may have utilized—or are still utilizing—sophisticated systems to pulverize your spirit into compliance with their self-seeking expectations, enforced through power, control, and exploitation. Unfortunately, even at this point in your development, your parents, siblings, and colleagues may still be critical and unsupportive of your remaining uniqueness and life direction. To know yourself, it is imperative that you review this history.

Unfortunately, it is likely that you, like most people, continue to criticize or judge yourself the same way you were criticized during your formative years. You pick up where others left off. You may have left the environment of your family of origin, yet because you are still programmed to think of yourself as a victim, you continue with abusive self-thought.

Bewildered, frustrated, and somewhat anxious or depressed, you probably blame yourself or others for your demise. Whose fault is it? Yours or others? Neither. It is the system's. It's about principles, not personalities.

Abusive society grinds your pride into your feet and fills the empty space with shame. Furthermore, an abusive societal system will produce an abusive result. It gets what it gives. A shame-based system, fortified with guilt tactics, displaces your self-worth and traps much of your spirit in your backpack.

Remember the exercise on page 13? The level at which you placed your hands defines or measures how much of your spirit and self-esteem you retain and how much you carry on your back.

Can we change society? Can we truly impact the next generation, much less the next seven generations?

We are, but slowly. To add momentum to this social revolution, we must begin with self.

Can we change and reconstruct self? Certainly. So let's get started.

This book has been designed and written to restore health and sacredness to your relationships, beginning with yourself. The purpose of this section is to begin healing your relationship with yourself. It encourages you to reach in your backpack, retrieve, and reclaim those parts of your spirit burdening your life. Only you can retrieve them to reconstruct yourself.

The formula is quite simple: *Add value* to self rather than *devalue* self.

What's the worst thing that will happen? You'll get too healthy, too happy? You'll become too accepting and content with yourself? You'll be contagiously healthy? Don't worry about it. You may just end up enjoying your uniqueness and come to value your personage. We hope that you'll become your own best friend. That's our goal. In the process, you will need to learn new constructive systems to replace your present destructive systems. As you add value to self, you add value to all others, to all future generations.

It is time to rediscover and redesign yourself. First, however, you must rediscover who you truly are, to know yourself. Know the depths of you, as the dolphin knows the sea. Know the height of you, as the eagle knows the sky. Know the breadth of you, as the winds know all directions. Know the secrets within you, as each stone knows Mother Earth.

It all begins and ends with yourself. And you begin and end with your identity. In other words, who are you? Do you really know yourself? How can you possibly *be* yourself if you don't really *know* yourself?

This next exercise will require time. If you do not have the time right now, make an appointment and reserve a quiet time for yourself.

Exercise

Please take out a piece of paper and, for the next ten minutes, allow yourself to write down thoughts about who you think you are. Give yourself permission to write from your heart, without distractions. Close the door or drive to a quiet place. Turn off the music, the TV, even the sound of your own voice. Just listen. Listen to the depth of you—your fears, loves, and grief—and reveal that. Listen to the height of you—your accomplishments, hopes, and dreams—and write that. Listen to the breadth of you—the directions of your life, the past, present, and future. Finally, listen to the silent secrets within, the inner workings and creations of your being. Reveal on paper what you *do* know about you. In this way, you claim those aspects that you may have kept hidden even from yourself. Do not censor yourself. Do not only write the things that you think are complimentary, nor only what you would like to change about yourself. Include it all. Be thorough. Allow your list to fill at least an entire page of paper. Please, take this time, now, to write down who you are. Do it in any way that feels comfortable to you, but be thorough.

What did you write? Did you write down the roles you take on? Did you write down the things you do? Did you write down the thoughts and emotions you experience?

If you didn't address the following questions, please do so now, on the back of your paper. What *is* your joy? Your children, work, flowers, music, God, your job, travel? What makes you sad? Missed opportunities, loved ones who have passed on, your character flaws, your job, stagnation, losses? Where are you headed? Nowhere, somewhere, anywhere? To college, to family, around the world, to a new job, to no job, to any job? What makes you happy? The first snowfall, sunset and sunrise, nature, your abilities, your family, learning, loving? What's important to you? What are your talents? Creating, being still, listening? They're from the spiritual world. What are your skills? Athletics, flying an airplane, or whipping up a batch of chocolate-chip cookies? They're from this world. What do you need? What do you want? A big house, a small house, quiet, activity, the ability to say no, the ability to say yes? How do you celebrate? How do you decorate yourself? What are the positive and negative aspects of yourself? What are your aspirations? What do you want to contribute? A piece of music, a loving family, a cleaner earth, a better day for someone sick, wealth for your grandchildren, a day of peace for all? What do you want to gather?

Do not be in a hurry to read what will come next. It will be here, when you are finished with your writing exercise. Give yourself the gift of time and presence. Our presence is the greatest gift we have to give. Find out who you are now.

Look over your list of ideas. Consider all that you have written in light of how it identifies you. Think in terms of roles and the activities in which you participate. Now reword your ideas into definitions of who you are: "I am a mother, daughter, lawyer, friend, cake decorator, musician; I am someone who enjoys nature, someone who sews, knits, runs."

Now take your ideas, one by one, and ask the question "Why?" "Why am I a friend, a mother, a teacher? Why do I play tennis, enjoy the outdoors, cook gourmet food? Why do I think about the things I think about? Why am I a singer, a writer, a comedian? Why do I need another person in my life? Why do I enjoy working with my hands?" Follow each idea back until you can go no further. Continue to ask *why* after each answer until you exhaust the *whys*. Each answer will contain the word *because,* which leads to the next *why*.

For example, you might write: "I enjoy writing because it is creative." Why is it creative? "It is creative because I am free to let go." Why are you free to let go? "I am free to let go because. . . ." In this manner, you will find the essence of who you are. This may take some time. Try to write at least three or four statements that most meaningfully identify who you are. Please, do this now.

———

Our guess is that you have found some very illuminating truths about who you are at your essence. The example above might continue like this: "I am free to let go because I trust. I trust because I feel safe inside." Perhaps you discovered that you are a child of nature. Maybe you only went back far enough to uncover intense feelings or a need for others. Try to go back as far as you possibly can: "I feel safe inside because it is a place where no one can enter. No one can enter because it is a sacred place." Perhaps you stopped at the mysteries that are unanswerable. Do not be afraid of your answers. Trust. Only you will hear your voice speak the truth. Give birth to who you are: "It is a sacred place because it is from the Creator. It is from the Creator because he or she created me. He or she created me because he or she loves me."

Wherever you end up, you will be closer to your essence than you were five minutes ago. Perhaps you remembered the love that you are. Perhaps you remembered you are a being who needs to experience this world. Love, truth, life, and the mystery of all are the yearnings of our spirit. Do not keep reflections such as these reserved only for moments of great joy or tragedy in your life. Reflect now so you can see who you are today. This may be your last day on this earth. Perhaps you discovered that you are a being who needs to give and receive love and light. Notice how all your answers deal with relationships—with yourself, others, the universe, or God. Relationships, the connections between this world and the next, are the most sacred of all.

We have a three-fold definition of the word *sacred:* "worthy of respect," "dedicated to or set apart for the worship of God," and "made or declared holy." *Holiness* refers to that which belongs to, is derived from, or is associated with a divine power. For some, the idea of considering you and your relationships as sacred is natural. Eastern religions and the spirituality of indigenous people, for example, see the sacred in everything. There is no "it"; all of life is God- or Creator-filled. For others raised with Western thinking, *sacred* may be reserved for a few places, things, and God him- or herself. However, even the traditional Christian sacraments point you to another truth. Think of the times people have said to you, "God bless you." Blessings are said to invoke divine favor upon you. Mother Teresa proclaimed: "Holiness is not the luxury of a few. It is everyone's duty: yours and mine." Logically, then, divine favor would most definitely be associated with or derived from a divine power. Holiness is its result. Whichever way you look at it, then, you and your relationships are sacred.

This is who you are. Sacred. That is who I am. Sacred.

Here, you and I are the same. In our unique voyage, we each journey to the same ocean. To the very beginning of you and to the very beginning of me. To the very end of you and to the very end of me. We are both sacred. In this, I am you; we are one within each other, a part of an enormous system.

Perhaps the question really is *what* are you? Maybe *what* you are is a composite of *why* you are. You are physical, mental, emotional, and, at your deepest level, spiritual. And what, then, is spirit? Worldwide wisdom supported by the laws of physics refers to spirit as an unchanging energy that cannot be destroyed—only transformed. Hence, life after death. Energy is vibration. Every living thing in the universe has a vibration. Everything is composed of vibrating molecules. Consider the vibrating elements that constitute the tree, the plant, the fish, the deer, the bear, and the turtle. Continue this exploration; consider the air, the fire, the water, and the mineral. All that we know of life has a spiritual vibration. Which vibration is more important? Probably none, since all life forms need one another for continued balance, equilibrium, and health. Each has their purpose and equal right to existence. Respect for all existence ensures the web of life will not be torn or polluted, guaranteeing futuristic equity for all species.

Throughout the ages, vibrations have been manifested or observed as tiny specks of light. Consider electrons, heat, color, and sound—even auras. Some are subtler than others. Some phenomena are easily seen, while others require a new vision in order to perceive what undeniably exists. The light you can see, feel, and experience within yourself, others, and the universe forms if you quiet yourself enough to experience it and if all distractions are eliminated. In fact, darkness, or an emptiness or openness, is needed. A new vision is needed, without distractions, in order to see what is already there. The northern lights are a spectacular view, but only at night. Atoms are visible, but only within the vast dark space that surrounds them. The light of others is recognizable, but only if we quiet ourselves down long enough to see them without distracting thoughts. Indeed, darkness better emphasizes the light.

Likewise, we must look within our darkness in order to see our light.

Consider that you are, at your deepest level, an indestructible light-form-vibration suspended in time, within a present body, with the ability to think and feel.

Consider, also, that you consist of more space than substance. In fact, according to some scientists, only .001 percent of what we perceive as real—what we cling to—is actually physical matter. Within each atom, there is 99.999 percent empty space.

Consider, the vast majority of who we are is nothingness! Given this reasoning, letting go of *one thousandth* of our existence—or dying—really shouldn't be a big deal!

Only when we come to know who we are, when our vision is clear at the deepest level, are we free to truly be ourselves. Ultimately, on our deathbeds, we will not be concerned with what we did, but rather with who we were and, ultimately, what we are—an expansion of our spirit.

When you are willing to look within, to see your dark emptiness without judgment, wishes, or borrowed eyes, then you will be able to see the truth. What is, is. The truth is that you are who you are. This is a vitally important concept to understand, for all that will follow rests on this very basic premise. You are you. Trust yourself.

Be Self

One of the first questions we may be asked when our journey here on earth ends is "Were you *you?*" Possibly all that is expected from you in this lifetime is for *you* to fully experience *who you are.*

As a vibrating being of light, you are the creation of your experiences, hopes, fears, and circumstances. *But even more than that, you are the creation of your spiritual journey.* Your spirit's journey is sacred. You are being provided with the nourishment that your spirit needs to come closer to God, to become able to hold a greater quantity of the Creator's energy within your spirit.

Soon enough we will leave our physical bodies here on this earthly plane and return home in our pure spirit form.

We will take nothing back home from this physical side, not even a berry that we ate that morning. What we take back home are our experiences. Therefore, live your life to the fullest, because the food of life is experience. Moreover, what other possible reason could there be for leaving the spirit world to come to the physical side, except to live life to the fullest? The reason it is called life is because we are to live it.

In order to live *your* life, you must be *you*. Not your mother's or father's expectation of whom you should be or become, but you. Not your siblings' or children's expectations of whom you should be, but you. Too often, each generation lives to fulfill the previous generation's expectations. No one ends up living his or her own life.

Recently, we heard of a woman who is planning her funeral. Even with the knowledge that she is living her last days, others are attempting to influence her decisions regarding what kind of funeral she should have. She has chosen to plan as she wishes, however. Will you wait until your last days to finally assert yourself?

Please take this time to consider whether or not you are living your life. Are you doing what *you* want to do? Do you express yourself in your own way? Do you experience life with your internal vision or do you constantly wonder how others see you and accommodate their expectations?

Just as it is vital that you distinguish between your life and another's, it is critical to understand what *being* is all about.

Being and *doing* are two entirely different states. Being refers to the ability to rest in one's own presence, to wear it like a loose robe. Sit on a stump and *be* with the world around you. Listen to music and *enjoy* the pleasure it gives you. *Experience* how it feels to walk, to laugh, to sit, to run, to eat, to see, to hear, to touch, to stop, to listen, to know, to question, to breathe, to honor, to just *be.*

You may recognize the people who have mastered this art of being. She is the one who instantly dances to the jazz on the radio. He is the one who chews his food with great enjoyment. They are the ones who smile easily, laugh often, sigh softly. They are the ones who pass this on to the next generation, then the next and the next. Their ease with life is felt sevenfold.

Can you just be? Today, look for ways in which you can stop your doing in order just to experience, observe, and enjoy the world around you and the world within you. Be a human being who is not caught up in doing.

Becoming involves both stillness and activity, both being and doing. Becoming is not only what you do. Becoming is what you allow to happen. Too often people think they are only valuable if they are *doing* something. Stopping life long enough to just *be* goes against cultural expectations that tie value to productivity. How can we truly know who we are (and then act on that knowledge) if we haven't taken the time to trust being in personal silence and stillness? Unfortunately, those of us who do not pause long enough, and often enough, to experience our own silence are unable to experience the necessary steps of knowing, being, and giving. Silence is the essence of the Creator.

Knowing is the prerequisite to doing. Once you have determined the essence of who you are, embracing your being, you are able to celebrate your life at a deeper level. Have you discovered what gives you such joy or bliss? If not, take this moment to discover what you do that causes you to lose track of time and, at the same time, makes you more you. (Here lies the distinction. Addictions may cause you to lose track of time, but they do not contribute to your authentic becoming.) Whatever it is, that is the path you need to follow. It is the way you lift your spirit. It is your personal form of spirituality.

Your spirit recognizes this and gives you hints that you are on the right path. Bliss, timelessness, effortlessness, contagious inspiration, movement, joy, creativity, epiphanies, and growth are keys to understanding your path. Your spirit is beyond time and space. What carries you beyond the shackles of the clock is the path to your becoming.

An acorn does not become a butterfly. An acorn becomes an oak tree. A caterpillar becomes a butterfly. One must be present with the moment in order for the becoming to happen. Similarly, a caterpillar does not *wish* to become a butterfly. Somewhere inside, it instinctively *knows* it will. It instinctively trusts itself and the universe to provide the transformation. It experiences being a caterpillar and follows the path to the inevitable transformation. Do you know that right now, at this moment, you, too, are in transformation? That somewhere inside *you* the knowledge of what you are to become exists? Trust that it does. Although transformation may not be recognizable each moment, transformation does occur and is seen eternally.

You must be willing to be who you are now in order to be who you will become. The path that engages your spirit is the path that will lead you to your destiny. Follow your heart.

You must first know yourself, in order to…

Believe in the possibilities of you, in order to…

Practice the choices that lead to…

Becoming who you are meant to be.

Your sacred relationship with yourself is about knowing, believing, practicing, and becoming. Personal choices and decisions can then be focused on a solid understanding of who you are and what you value. Remember that even inactivity and indecision are decisions.

Listen to these words of becoming from our book *Earth Dance Drum.* In metaphorical language, understanding may slip in.

> Flow with time, but be present with each moment. Consider the vibration of the hummingbird's wings. Which of its flutter is flight? Is flight the past fluttering of its wing? Or is flight the next flap of the wing? Come to see that flight is all of this. Transcend and flow with time, yet be present with the moment. Like all of the winged, in order to transcend, we, too, must be in movement. We must vibrate. Truth after truth after truth reveals itself at each fluttering of our spiritual wings. Like the gradual shading of blue to green, we become, we live the transformations. It is as though we are in a cocoon within a cocoon within a cocoon. The more truths we experience, the more we are set free in colorful flight. Always in movement, the different levels of consciousness we experience lead us to the next level. This is how we come to soar.
>
> During your spiritual metamorphosis, you will remember your past and greet your future. In your transformation, you will honor your ancestors and leave a legacy. You will grow to appreciate your mistakes and your pain because it was the fluttering that kept you in flight. In your flight, you will understand the connectedness.
>
> Do it to become it.

Give Self

What you choose to practice, you are choosing to become. It is that simple. That is your ultimate gift to the universe. That is your gift to the seventh generation. If you are able to practice both stillness and doing, your journey will be clear. Your joy will show the way. Trusting the process of becoming is vital. From here, you have much to give. It will be contagious, as your bliss will inspire others. Practice new thinking of how your present actions and decisions will enhance the next seven generations. That's how you ingrain new behavioral systems.

Giving of ourselves implies that there is something to give. What do you have to give to others that is truly and uniquely yours? Money and material things belong ultimately to the material world. Since we are spiritual beings encased in physical bodies, what we truly have to give can only be that which is ours to give: Our presence. Our love. Our life. Our flesh. Our thoughts. Our emotions. Our attention.

Consider, right now, how you could give the gift of your presence today. How will you listen? What love can you share? When? For whom would you be willing to sacrifice your life? For what? Why? What truths in your keeping ask to be revealed? How can you educate? How will you share your emotions? What will you attend to? Will you be here, now?

As you truly understand and embrace that this type of giving is all that we really have to give another, then all other physical aspects of giving will be more natural and unconditional.

What is your talent? Share it with others. What is your strength? Give it to others. What is your passion? Reveal it to others. What is your understanding? Teach it to others. What is your love? Give it to others. What is your knowledge? Pass it on from generation to generation, preferably in story form, as values are best sustained within verbal pictures of storytelling.

You will no longer give to receive. But the irony is that you will receive. You will become more fully you and more genuinely you in the process of knowing, being, and giving. The seventh generation will be gifted when you gift yourself.

Chapter Two

Listening Awareness

Life will inevitably ask us to stop, if not today, then eventually. Consider yourself, stopped in this moment: your thoughts stopped, your emotions stopped, your body stopped. It is not easy. As soon as we stop our bodies, our thoughts run a marathon. As soon as we stop our thoughts, our bodies find something to do. As soon as we stop our emotions, we feel lost. No wonder stopping will be the last thing we do on this earth. It is a difficult task, stopping. Yet this challenge will come, if not today, then eventually.

Stopping asks us to listen. When this stopping occurs for you, what will you hear? Listening asks us to attend. What will you experience at the closing moment? Soak in the experience of stopping now. It is in our silence that we come to know our spiritual identity. We must shed our physical identity—our movements, thoughts, and feelings—momentarily to clearly embrace our spiritual identity.

Many people would rather wait for the moment of ultimate transformation than deal with the possibilities of transformation here on earth. It takes time, it takes attention, it takes us away from this world. We cling to our lives here on earth. However, truly, as spiritual guides have echoed, those who learn to die learn to live. Letting go is required in life. We all will experience not just one, but many losses in our lifetimes. We all experience loss throughout our days here on earth. Learning how to be with death, at all levels, experiencing the stages of grief—yes even that of letting go of the moment—ultimately prepares us for the final journey.

Understanding loss and accepting loss are key to receiving all that life has to give. Pope John XXIII once stated, "The shadow better emphasizes the light." Indeed, one is needed for the other. Life cannot fully exist without its counterpart of death. Death is the ultimate experience of life. We are born to die. But what we experience between conception and death will calibrate the expansion of our spirit and measure the spiritual growth we have experienced in our lifetime.

Stopping is a form of loss. When we slow down enough to actually experience moments of stopping, we have let go of the life to which we are accustomed. We stop clinging to life and die a minideath.

Gaining this awareness grows out of intention, however. It must begin with the choice to slow down. Even slowing down will give you intimations of stopping, and the quality of your life will dramatically improve.

Awareness is thus all of this: slowing down, listening and attending. It requires mindfulness, focused attention, and deliberate *being* instead of doing.

Slowing down, listening to your body and your heart, is like the bubbles that form in a babbling brook. Our life is often so busy, so hectic, so full of movement and distraction that the bubbles of nothingness are never attended to. Instead, we see the movement, we hear the rush of life, we feel the cold and warmth, but we rarely experience how it feels to float above the movement of the brook encased in a bubble of spirit, to become one with all, part of the movement, yet somehow detached from the course of obstacles and urgency.

Here, in stillness, the bubbles stay undisturbed for a time, even though what moves beneath may be turbulent. With spiritual awareness, we, too, can remain unchanged—experiencing our nature of nothingness—although what we experience in the physical dimension is movement, sound, and passion. Eventually, the bubbles burst back into the brook and air to be part of the stream and the sky, only to reemerge after something deep inside the river moves them back to the top of consciousness.

There are many ways to arrive at this experience, just as there are many reasons why bubbles emerge. Become the bubble of the invisible in order to participate more fully in the visible world.

Slow Down

Can you stop? This may sound like a very ridiculous question, for in theory, everyone knows what *stop* means. "Simon Says" taught us this at an early age. But if you are like most people, truly stopping is a rare occurrence. Listen to a Zen teaching: "If you are stopping now, then stop. If you are looking for a time that you will finish, there will never be a time that you will finish." Yes, to varying degrees, most people can stop their bodies for a time. External stopping (except in some medical conditions), like playing statue as a child, is more of a matter of willpower and mind control. Internal stopping is about intention.

Putting on the brakes of our mind is far more difficult than it would seem. Try it, right now. Stop.

What happened? Did you experience the split second of no thoughts only to be immediately brought back to internal doing, with various thoughts floating in and out of your consciousness? If so, you have begun the journey to understanding slowing down.

We would like to suggest that there are many ways to arrive at this stillness. Spiritual practices include following your breath, ceremony, prayer, and meditation. In fact, humming to achieve internal vibration can be very soothing. Humming vibrates your inner world and resonates your spirit. All of these practices can help us to slow down and stop. They have endured for thousands of years.

However, we would suggest that slowing down is perhaps the first step in our journey to stillness. Slowing down needs to be a prerequisite to spiritual practices like breathwork, prayer, meditation, and ceremony. Our culture has conditioned us to want things *now*. That has become our nature. A quick trip through a drive-through meditation clinic would appeal to many. Immediate gratification and a desire to cling to the remaining moments of each day continue to haunt us. Trying to shove a thirty-minute breathing exercise into a hectic day is like painting a turtle with water paints and then putting it back into the water. The results do not last.

Indeed, it's more like slamming on the brakes—as a result, you could be thrown. A gradual slowing down may best prepare you for listening awareness.

Our environment can assist us in slowing down. Ceremonies, tribal or spiritual, are deliberate and often help to slow us down. Designing daily or weekly ceremonies of your own can help to slow you down internally.

Take a walk. Don't power walk, not with this exercise in mind, at least. Walk slowly and deliberately. The farther away from the distractions of others you go, the better. If you can go out in nature, you will more easily slow down. Notice. See the sunlight as it filters through the leaves. Watch the flight of a flock of birds. Experience the touch of a caterpillar against your skin. Be present with the song of the forest. Listen. Hear the wind, the waves, the birds, the chipmunks, the branches, and the ice breaking free from the branches. Experience your body. Feel the heat, the cold, the pain, the ache, the sweetness, the strength after a run, and the forest-air-medicine as it enters your lungs. Experience your thoughts. Follow the repetitions, the dance, the wanderings of your mind. Experience yourself.

Notice how our elders walk. They have discovered this secret, even if their bodies demand it of them. They walk with presence. They notice. They have slowed down. Watch an infant study her mother. The very act of seeing is slow and complete, as infants are still close to the other side and embrace all symmetry. Balance, inherent to symmetry, is recognized.

Do your housework or yard work at a slower pace. Notice your body: how your hands move, your legs work, your back feels. Extend and contract your muscles and feel them as though for the first time. Take your time. Do not rush to get to the next chore. Be with the activity you are working on now. Be here, now. Feel the bubbles in the sink, the earth in your hands, the sun on your back, the snow on your face, the rain on your skin. Whatever the weather, whatever the time of day, *slow down.*

Eat your next meal with deliberate attention. Thank the carrot for giving its life so you can live.

Practice right now by selecting something to eat. Chew and experience the texture and taste before you swallow. Smell before you bite. Reach and notice the food before you smell. Feel the food go down your throat and fill your stomach before you reach. Slow down your chewing, tasting, and swallowing.

As you slow down, your thoughts will slow down. The mind/body connection will assist you in internal slowing down. It is really quite simple. Deliberately slow down! Find ways throughout your day to practice this. Easy does it! Where there is easiness, there is no uneasiness.

Your Body Is Smarter than Your Mind

Despite the fact that a disproportionate amount of space supports the existence of our material world, the physical realm is the context in which we live and learn. Although we are not our bodies, we are given bodies through which we experience life.

The .001 percent connects to the other 99.999 percent to make a whole. In this connection, our bodies are thereby the communicators or the liaisons between nothingness and somethingness. Listen to your body; there are messages awaiting your attention.

Our bodies, according to some traditions, are sacred temples. What is housed within must be honored. We must take care of the temple to ensure the health of its occupant.

Have you ever experienced the urge to run? To drink milk? To sleep? To get fresh air? To eat an apple? These internal urges originate from the body, not the mind. Not many people have a mind that *wants* to run. In fact, most of us could think of many reasons *not* to run: I'm tired. I'm getting older. I'd rather press the snooze button. There's a good show on TV. But many people have a body that wants to run and dance and walk and sleep. Cravings are sometimes the body's way to communicate that something is lacking. Crave a banana? You need potassium. Crave an ice cream cone? You're probably lacking calcium. Listen to your body to find out what it is that you need. Crave sleep? Then sleep!

Your body knows more than you think it does, and it will continue to urge you to do what is necessary for balance and health. If you do not listen to your body, your body will make you listen. It will get sick and make you do the things it needs. As the adage goes, "If you don't take time for health now, you'll take time for sickness later."

People think of medicine as something to take after you get sick, to relieve symptoms. But if you don't want to get sick, you need to take "medicine" *before* you get sick.

What are real medicines? Smelling flowers is medicine. When was the last time you smelled a flower? Eating healthy foods is medicine. What did you eat today? Crying and laughing are great medicines. Have you cried recently? Do you allow yourself to cry? Have you laughed until your gut hurt? Exercise is great medicine. What do you do regularly to exercise your body? Art is medicine. What literature, music, visual art, or movies have you voluntarily delved into lately? Dancing is medicine. When was the last time you let loose? Tapped your foot? Sang a song? Creative exploration is medicine. What ways do you creatively express yourself? Perhaps one of the greatest medicines of all is nature. Simply breathing in good, clean air is medicine. Do you know what it smells like? Can your nose identify wild blueberries growing nearby? Can you smell a river? Watch what you put in your mouth, then play, relax, laugh, cry, have fun. Engage yourself in a balanced lifestyle. These are all true medicines.

Watch animals. Animals, more closely in tune with their bodies, will naturally eat what they need to remain healthy. A deer eats medicines from the forest. A dog will chew on grass. A bird will select gravel to digest its food. We can learn a lot from watching animals. And please, don't forget, we *are* animals. We may not have fins and feathers, but we, too, are of the animal kingdom.

Too often, in all our wisdom, we screw things up. Consider college campuses. Architects lay concrete sidewalks from building to building. Students come along, find better routes, and begin making their own trails, often not using sidewalks at all. Rather than letting the students (or the body) create paths where they need to be, the "mind" of the campus decides on the path, hoping the students will follow. This is backward. Likewise, we need to let our bodies tell our minds what works and doesn't work. Trust your body. Your body wants what is best for you. Your body even knows what type of tears to secrete depending on the circumstances.

You need to let your body, not your head, make your schedule.

Your body knows when to eat, when to drink, when to rest and exercise. Listen to your body, and your body will take good care of you. Forget all the guidelines about how much sleep you *should* get; after all, we are individuals with individual needs. Eight hours for one person is not enough for another, or it may be too much for someone else.

In addition to following the dictates of your body to create a balanced lifestyle, there are times when you must heed the life stressors that beg for your attention. Have you ever experienced extreme tension after an arduous commute to work? Day after day, the stress of such a drive builds up and creates a state of distress within. Do long hours at work compromise your ability to maintain balance? Although stress is inevitable in our world, the way you respond to stress can provide a creative opportunity. What changes is your body begging you to make? Take the time to listen and become aware of all the messages your body is giving you.

Distinguish between positive stress and distress. Good stress promotes creativity and production. Negative stress actually diminishes our abilities and erodes our internal balance. This subjection to physical or mental strain will take its toll. Become aware of negative stress in your daily life. Do your shoulders ache at night? What are you holding in there? Persistent stress leads to distress. Do your hands hold the day's stressors? Memories are stored in your body, and a good massage will work out the memories. Pay attention to the body memories, as they may be keys to eliminating stress and promoting balance in your life.

Your mind can win, for a while, insisting that what you are experiencing is only normal. Eventually, however, your body will demand to be heard. Listen. Be aware. When you truly listen to your body and realize that changes are necessary, your commitment to change will invite the universe to support your efforts. Doors begin to open and alternatives become available.

Work to listen more closely to your body. Unhealthy indulgence does not come from your body. Those are more likely psychological urges and pacifications your injured spirit wants in order to medicate the pain. Natural balance is the way of the body. Balance is about preventing and healing pain. When your body wins, you win.

Listen to Your Heart

What is it that you yearn to do? What have you put on the back burner, waiting for the right time to bring it forward? What makes you happy?

Just as listening to your body, rather than your mind, takes some getting used to, so does listening to your heart. As the body communicates, the heart senses. In our society, we are expected to think, not feel, or at least govern our feelings with solid, rational thought. However, how many of us, really, are more concerned with our thoughts than our hearts? Who among us will be more concerned with thoughts, rather than feelings, at the time of death? Ultimately, it is your heart that indicates the quality of your life. The heart, ultimately, is the sensor of our life path or spiritual journey. The heart knows and lets us know whether we are on the right path, whom we need to be with, where we need to go, what we need to do. Be true to yourself: follow your heart.

Do you listen to your heart? Do you slow down long enough to be aware of the music of your heart? As with your body, your heart will not tolerate being neglected for long. Unhappiness is the result of a heart neglected. Unhappiness is the signal that *you* need to change. Are you happy? If not, why not? You probably already know why. Please take this time to acknowledge and verbalize your unhappiness.

Unhappiness is distinct from grief. Grief is sublime in its beauty for the totality of love felt for another, or for what has been lost. Grief is transforming and transitory, as it leads one to a new place of understanding. Yes, it is possible to be momentarily happy while grieving another. When your heart remembers a loved one, a smile may come to your lips. When you honor the one you love, can that not balm your ache with its tenderness? When you silently connect with the spirit of the one you love, can that not give you a sense of comfort and beauty? As you can love someone in his or her absence, so can happiness emit from your heart, as his or her spirit resides there. Indeed, happiness lives in the heart and is neighbor to grief.

Happiness comes from following the precepts of your heart. Happiness is not glee, giddiness, or even passion. Happiness is your heart fulfilled. It is possible to fill one's heart to overflowing. Have you ever experienced such a state of delight? Nothing comes close to this sweet nectar, the memory of which can be returned to in times of pain as a source of comfort. Happiness is of this world. Bliss comes from the spirit world. Joy has a foot in both worlds.

As you become more accustomed to slowing down and listening to the world both inside and outside you, you may find silence the best sound of all. You may even begin to crave silence as you once craved distractions. Try listening amid the noisy streets on a typical working day. Now try listening within the dark borders of a forest. Although masters can listen wherever they are, you may want to begin where silence is most easily accessible.

Find the places in your world where you can shut the door and be alone with yourself. In this place, your heart will tell you the secrets that it has been longing to share. In this space of aloneness, you may even find more of who you are and what you need to be. You can be alone and not lonely. Trust the silence, for the heart is home here.

Here is the place in which the seven generations are heard, including the first generation: yourself. Trust the silence; trust your heart and body. Trust your being and becoming and giving. Come to know yourself, and you will come to glimpse beyond yourself. First, with the trust of the universe on your side, come home to you. Come within yourself to your spiritual home within your heart, where your spirit and your Creator's spirit interconnect within silence. How peaceful, how joyful, how serene! Ensure this tranquility for the next seven generations. It's all about experiencing self and thereby becoming a guardian for future generations—truly an honorary commission.

PART TWO

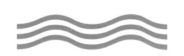

TRANSFORMING AND TRANSCENDING SELF

Chapter Three

So Many Choices

We grow into the seventh generation. For good or bad, the seventh generation ultimately reflects the changes of each previous generation. You are a mirror to the future. The seventh generation is a consequence of either previous attempts at growth or previous contentment with the status quo. To embrace the potential of ultimate betterment of your world, you must come to realize that growth will only occur within personal transformation and transcendence. Personal burgeoning not only beautifies the future, but also offers a soothing scent for today.

Transformation and transcendence have always paved the road that leads to serenity. Transformation refers to your ability to change and embrace change. Transformation, like the water cycle, is not about being someone different, but rather being who you really are in different forms. As ice is water is vapor, so are the extensions of yourself awaiting discovery. In other words, be true to yourself.

Transcendence refers to your ability to go beyond the ordinary to experience life. To transcend, you must be willing to open up your powers within. You must become aware. For if you are not aware, are you truly alive? To transcend what keeps you down, you must be willing to reach up. It is not just something that happens to you. Rather, you must participate in your own transcendence. You are the maker of yourself.

Are you willing to take responsibility for your own future? Are you able to let go of the past? Can you release the justifications and rationalizations that form the concrete reasoning behind why you are the way you are? Let go of excuses. Release the reasons. Do not cling to the past! Can you be someone who enjoys the jump? Can you let go and experience the moment in between? In-between space is the basis of all fear, but also the space of change.

In between known worlds, you may find yourself without footing, foreground, or background. It is here in this space of nothingness that you will truly grow. Ironically, you will come to appreciate the place of egolessness that exists inside you. To experience life, you must experience loss. To become who you are meant to be, you must let go. Oftentimes, this is the hard part that keeps you stuck. Choices need to be made.

Do you remember entering the candy store as a youngster with a dime in your pocket and marveling at all the choices? Can you recall those exciting smells? Lemon drops, chocolate stars, root beer barrels, caramels, candy corn, and so much more! But inevitably, did you always select the same candy? Was it because you were afraid to spend your money on something you weren't sure would bring you satisfaction? Or did you just know which candy was the one for you? Our guess is that you did indeed know your taste-bud preferences. Kids seem to know.

Unfortunately, as we grow into adulthood, choices seem to be less about knowing as they are about not knowing. Comfort and familiarity lead us to the same choices day after day, year after year. In fact, fear of the unknown seems to grow with age, unless we embrace the mystery within the fear. Again, clinging to the familiar keeps us from venturing forth and taking risks. In other words, we remain stuck. If nothing changes, then nothing changes.

Contrast someone who is simply old with the genuine under-standing and wisdom of an elder. The older our respected elders get, the more *they* respect what they do not understand. They are more willing to "not know." Respect begets respect.

Many people, however, remain stuck, if not comfortable, with the way they always do things. They are unwilling to try something new. This becomes the legacy for the next genera-tions. Even a new recipe may seem a terrible risk. "What if I don't like it?" A new haircut, a new philosophy, a new vision of oneself is simply out of the question. Being exposed to different cultures is threatening to some, as people mistakenly equate dif-ferences with an attack of the way they have been brought up. Differences are not right or wrong. They are simply differences. Unfortunately, multicultural exposure, to some, is like mutiny against the way things always have been and "should" be. It may also become a loyalty issue to our parents and others who raised us. Differences may threaten the idea of who we are. Unfortunately, those who push away diversity push away life itself. The mystery is never therefore honored, influencing future generations as well to push differences away. Life without diver-sity may become boringly bland, and we, too, become boring.

You can justify and rationalize like any "good" adult and thereby never expand your comfort zone—your province of pre-dictability. Indeed, here you reign: comfortable, secure, and unchanging.

This chapter is about recognizing the differences between healthy and unhealthy risks, as well as distinguishing between authentic preferences that engage your spirit and entrapments that hinder further spiritual and personal growth.

Prepare yourself for the journey. You are beginning to look down the path of life-darkness that will lead you into the light. It requires only one step at a time, one moment at a time, one breath at a time. The awareness of who you are will accentuate the shadows, to be sure, yet the challenge of who you are becoming will excite your spirit as it awaits your transformation. Your spirit enjoys transcendence.

You hold the key to the choices you make. It is the key to happiness. There are, indeed, so many choices. Are you aware of the possibilities that await your recognition? There's a lot of candy in the store of life! So fill your bag until your potential has actualized! Life is all about choices and actions.

Each day, you use your free will to respond to life, consider options, and make decisions. Each moment, you create your future. Each moment, you release the past. Each moment, you may choose to live to the best of your ability.

Free Will, Our Most Precious Gift

Free will is our most precious spiritual gift and resource. It's behind all personal choices and decisions, which are influenced by how we think and feel. Within each of us is the profound ability to create our outer existence. Yet even more astounding is our ability to create an inner existence that cannot be manipulated from the outside. Even those in the death camps in World War II realized their perpetrators could not invade this interior. What you hope, what you are passionate about, what you feel about yourself and the world cannot be assaulted by others. Free will is beyond the physical realm. The only people who can shackle our spirit are us.

You create each moment of each day and decide how you will live it *now*. Abraham Lincoln said, "People are just about as happy as they want to be." Happiness begins with our expectations and how we choose to use our free will.

People feel about as good as they want to because they, and they alone, determine all their emotional responses based on their thoughts and beliefs, which ultimately determine their feelings and consequent actions. There's rarely any reason to feel bad, unless you *choose* to feel bad or manufacture the reason. Your interpretations of facts, your thoughts and beliefs, beget your emotional responses. If you don't like the way you feel, then change your perspective.

Free will abides within your spirit. Indeed, many believe that, of free will, we decided to come to this earth to experience the parents and life circumstances that we were given. Could it be that we chose these circumstances as a means to spiritual growth, knowing before coming to this dimension that life here would be hard or painful? Are we here to expand our spiritual capacity? Perhaps this is so. Perhaps not.

But even considering this possibility forces us to look at our life from a totally different frame of reference. Indeed, this is a very healthy way to look at life, for in doing so, we give up the victim role, choosing to look at the circumstances of life and learn from them rather than being controlled by them.

We invite you to look at your life in this way: view all other events and circumstances as not happening *to* you, but rather happening *with* your permission and even *for* your growth.

This change in spiritual perspective has the potential to change everything! No longer are you a helpless victim, but a participant in life. The way you choose to respond to your life conditions will influence personal accountability. You will begin to see every event and circumstance as potentially meaningful. Inside each tragedy will be hidden a lesson or opportunity. Each character flaw will burgeon personal growth. Buried under layers of resentment, the power to forgive will emerge.

Your view on life, then, is the first aspect of free will that can potentially liberate you. Your intrinsic view will become your extrinsic view. If you want to change your external circumstance, you need to change your internal circumstance. This change will harvest new responses to previous reactions. For example, we continue to change the way we view uncharted challenges. Visualizing the outcome gives direction, with the effort usually resulting in something close to, equal to, or even better than what we originally imagined. Whether it be an artistic piece, a new program, or a project, it must first begin with an internal vision of the expected outcome.

Free will goes beyond *thinking* and *believing* and inspires *doing*. This is probably not the way you usually think of free will. Free will is about discipline and doing. However, we suggest you first use your free will to determine your course before revving up your engine.

With a new framework through which to view life, you are free to act upon your values and beliefs (addressed in more detail in chapter 4). Free will does exactly as the concept implies. You are *free*. And you *will*. Free will begets a new way of viewing yourself, for with every action we take, we change. Your body changes after you eat an apple. Your body changes after a good hard run. Your body changes without the proper amount of sleep. Your mind changes after learning something new. Your mind changes after experiencing an *aha* or insight. Your mind changes with the loss of a loved one. You are never the same. You are constantly being renewed, sculptured, and chiseled.

Therefore, your free will is the springboard to who you want to be now . . . and now . . . and now. The springboard is your intent.

Even we, as authors, are changing as we write and read these words. We will never be the same. Indeed, we are using our free will to trust the universe to provide the words that are yet to come. We come to the pen, paper, and computer with an open mind. Placing our fingers around the pen and upon the keys, we trust the universe to provide. It always does. We don't have to wait. The words are always there, waiting for us to open up to

them in order for them to flow through us. We are but a frequency in this process. Vibration after vibration after vibration
forms a frequency, a flowing momentum.

What can you open up to? It must first begin with trust, and
trust emerges from a state of free will. Willingly allow the universe to open doors for you. Willingly ask the universe to teach
you. Willingly open to the wonder of life—*your* life. With your
free will, become new. Transform and transcend self.

The secret is to remove whatever it is that is blocking this
energy flow. What are you blocked with? Anger, resentment,
guilt, remorse, fear? Let go and let the energies of the universe
automatically fill the void of openness.

Positive Begets Positive, Negative Begets Negative

Your choices, really, are simple: They are either positive choices that promote spiritual growth or negative choices that lead to
spiritual decay or stagnation. Everything you choose to think, do,
believe, practice, and expect is either helpful or harmful.

Incredibly, we rarely consider all of our moment-to-moment
choices in this light, as it seemingly requires a lot of emotional
and mental energy. We generally reserve this type of analyzing
for the big decisions in life: a new job, marriage, children, economic decisions. Of course, we should. However, please consider
the choices you are making every day in view of whether they are
positive or negative, proactive or destructive, helpful or hurtful.

The effort you invest in these daily decisions may well make
your other major decisions seem effortless or even nonexistent.
With each decision, you lay the groundwork that leads up to the
"big" ones. Some problems may never even arise; for example,
if you are physically fit and eat healthy to begin with (as a result
of small, proactive decisions made every day), you might never
have to deal with the bigger decisions that arise from a major
health problem.

Negative begets negative, and positive begets positive. All you need to do is answer a very simple question with each decision, no matter how small: Is this a positive choice or a negative choice? Is this helpful or hurtful? Identifying the potential of each thought, belief, action, or nonaction is the first step in making proactive changes in your life. Now, try to imagine the consequences of each decision as its tendrils reach out to one generation, then another. We hurt or help not just this generation (me); we hurt or help all future generations (we).

Exercise

For the next exercise, write down as many of today's thoughts, beliefs, actions, expectations, and nonactions as you can. Brainstorm a list and be as thorough as possible. Identifying actions will be easiest. Please, do this now.

Please look over your list. Identify an irrational, destructive, or unhealthy belief. You know at some level what is unhealthy. Write that belief in a complete statement form. On a separate piece of paper, write a replacement belief that is healthy, proactive, and productive. Now crush up, throw away, or burn your first destructive belief and retain the new healthy replacement belief. In addition, write your new belief on one side of an index card or a cloth poker chip. On the opposite side, write practical ways to achieve it. Carry this with you or place in a prominent spot to remind you. Do it to become it. Place the chip in your pocket, so that every time you reach in, touching it will remind you of your new commitment to self. Or tape your card to a wall, mirror, or refrigerator, so that every time you look up you remember. Repetition of new behavior extinguishes old behavior.

Look over your list once again. How many of the things that you thought about, did, expected, or believed were actually something *new* for you? We tend to repeat the same thought patterns, expectations, beliefs, and actions over and over, day after day, introducing few, if any, new ideas or actions into our lifestyle. We form a comfortable zone of dysfunction, so to speak, and bask in its negativity.

Now, looking at your list, what percent of the repetitious patterns were actually good for you? What percent were negative? This is vital.

Positive choices will lead to positive outcomes. Negative choices will lead to negative outcomes. Choose positive over negative. If you don't, you are doomed to repeat the same mistakes over and over. *If we always do what we've always done, we'll always get what we've always "got" and if nothing changes, nothing changes.*

Now, consider what you could do differently. How could you eliminate and replace the negative? Try something new that is also positive! In this way, you are ensuring positive results while expanding your personal view, your world view, and perhaps your spiritual view as well.

Be the seed in the wind; journey the currents to new environments and gather nourishment for you to grow anew. Notice how what you do, risk, and become influences your children's expectations for themselves. This cannot be overstated. We influence our children in ways we'll never know. Silently, as you travel to new places, so do your children catch the current of your journey. You leave a trail.

Options and Potential

You authored your psychological programming to survive your childhood family and environment. What makes you think this programming serves you well today in another family, circumstance, and environment?

Do you have any idea of your own personal potential and options? We are beings with unlimited potential, ability, and promise. Our problem often lies in not being able to recognize that we actually have options. Too often, we tell ourselves we don't have a choice: "I *have* to go to work. I *can't* do this or I *can't* do that." What we are really saying is, "I *choose* to go to work. I *won't* do this or I *won't* do that."

I can't means *I won't!* If you tell yourself, "I can't," you're right. If you tell yourself, "I can," you're right. Intent, intent, intent!

We always have options. There are many careers to choose from. In fact, many American workers make career changes midlife. As heard in a recent movie, there's nothing to change in the very beginning of life, and at the end of life it's generally too late. It only makes sense that the middle of our life is the best time you can truly make changes.

As you confront your predictability patterns, you need options. Do you know your options? What ten things do you want to do in your life? What experiences do you crave? Think about all the things you have once considered but perhaps dismissed as impossible. What do you want to contribute before you return to the spirit world? Everyone understands something that no one else understands. What tracks do you want to leave for others to follow for the next seven generations?

Exercise

To go a step further, please consider the following: Name five things you could do, right now, instead of the job you have.

———

What did you write down? Was it a difficult task? The more you were able to list—with the least amount of anxiety—the more options you see for yourself. Notice that we didn't say, "Name five things you could do right now that will give you the exact same economic and social rewards (or stress)."

Options imply differences. Too often, we are hesitant to step out of the comfort zone to which we are accustomed. Change requires change. Change is not always comfortable. Change is not always easy. Change is often scary! Change is mysterious. However, change can also be exciting! Change can even be fun.

Expect your options to require something of you. You are not just a passenger along for a ride. You must steer your own course and acknowledge the changes *you* must go through in order to experience the results of change.

You also have many options regarding how you think and see the world. You can see the world as boring. Or you can see the world as bubbling with exciting possibilities, and you can see yourself as a whole pool of possibilities. Again, it's *your* choice.

In the voice of Gina's sixth-grade students, "There's always another way! Face your fears! Believe! Have fun!" In the voice of our children, *hear* the wisdom of the ages. There are so many options for us to choose from! It's up to us to face our fears and believe. To make it so. To make life fun. If life doesn't contain fun, what's the point?

Exercise

If God materialized before your eyes, right now, what would she or he tell you *about you?* Write the one sentence God would say, now.

———

Perhaps you wrote something to this effect: "You are my beloved creation, filled with all the potential of all my creation." Or God might say, "Just hang in there; that's life's greatest secret."

Whatever you wrote, it came from your spiritual wellspring. This is where you need to return in order to discover your own potential. Trust yourself and the Creator to provide the vision you need to make the next positive choice.

Your potential is already stored in your spiritual genetic makeup. You already exist completely as you are meant to exist, in your spirit. Your spirit is complete. Our human frailties, preoccupations, and blockages prevent us from fully experiencing what is already there.

It's time to open your spiritual eyes to the truth of who you are. Go back to your discovery in chapter 1. You are a spiritual being who needs to give and receive love and light. You need to leave a legacy. You are a vital component to all sacred relationships. Consider your options after contemplating this truth.

Finally, list five things you could do right now instead of reading this book. Perhaps you could be with your daughter or son, ride your bike, take a walk, paint a picture, experience life. This book will be here. Will your son, daughter, granddaughter, grandson, husband, wife, mother, father, sister, brother be there? The greatest gift we can give anyone is our presence. Know your options and choose wisely. We can wait for you. Can they?

Decisions and Actions

What did you decide to do? We hope you chose wisely and realized that every decision you make leads to another. We want you to read this book. We also wish that you spend your time wisely, for every decision is connected to consequences. Some consequences are immediate. Some turn up days, weeks, months, even years later.

Be open to what is. Every moment presents you with endless possibilities. You need to determine which is the best choice for each moment. Reading this book is a good choice, but not when your son needs you. Sitting down with this reading may be a better choice if you find yourself giving, giving, giving and never having a moment for your own personal development. Balance your life.

Determine and act upon your inner voice. We know deep inside what we need to do. Really, it is not a mystery.

Too often, people ignore their internal voice and try to persuade themselves that what they've decided to do is really the best decision. Only later do they find out that they missed an opportunity. What can you learn? How can you simultaneously help your body and connect with a loved one? How about taking that walk? Playing? What do you *know* is the right thing to do now? You know it, so do it!

This is a critical point in developing a relationship with yourself. You must know yourself so completely that when you act upon your beliefs and values, you confidently make the right choice. Be true to yourself. Once you have acted, there is no need to go back.

Still, *you are responsible for your actions.* It is as simple as that. Only *you* get the credit or the blame. Learn from the voices of those who have made mistakes and live lives of regret. Regret, like anything else in life, is a continuum of severity.

While working in a nursing home, Gina learned a powerful lesson from two different residents. One, although living with dementia, lived every day in her memory in glorious connection with her loved ones. Believing her already-deceased family members were coming to visit, she prepared for each day with internal delight. Another resident, although completely cognizant of time and place, was filled with resentments and regret and was bitter about life.

Which fate would you choose? That of the first resident, completely in a bliss she created for herself by her obvious actions of love? Or the second? Which would matter more: not to know of time and place, or not to know love?

Our mental state reflects our moment-by-moment decisions and actions. What is your mental state reflecting? If you want to change the reflection on the lake, plant something new on the shoreline.

Your time and focus is very much an investment. You must choose where, when, and how you will invest yourself.

Depositing your effort and time in only one area will inevitably put a strain on another area of your life.

Who are you? You are a being who needs to give and receive love and light. What can you do to give love to yourself right now? Are you a human being or are you a human doing?

In all that you choose and do, remember your options, your perspectives, your potential, and your ability to freely create your moments. You are the maker, and the possibilities are endless.

CHAPTER FOUR

Redesign and Redirect

Can you envision yourself the way God sees you: perfectly yourself, fully experiencing life and contributing to the world, in complete alignment with your spirit? Much of what you are about to embark on must begin with your vision of yourself. You have the knowledge of who you are at your deepest level, a new ability to slow down and listen to life's messages, and full awareness of your potential and options. Prepare to engage in the hard work of becoming your destiny. This is where the beginning ripples inevitably reach out beyond self to the shores of all future generations. What you do or don't do ultimately has a ripple effect throughout the universe.

Chapter 4 is dedicated to guiding you through a redesign and redirection of your life experiences. You are still reading this book because either you are aware of the deficiency or difficulties that you continue to experience—due to past life experiences—or you are seeking to expand your growth. Although you are not responsible for getting knocked down in life, you *are* responsible for picking yourself back up. It's time to get up and get on. Get up, dust yourself off, and get on with the life experience.

You have a chance at a second lifetime. Come to see yourself as the artistic perfection Michelangelo saw hidden in the block of granite. All that you need to do is chisel away all that is *not* you. By doing this, you will, in effect, reclaim those parts of you that have been placed in your invisible backpack. You will return to yourself. By becoming open, honest, direct, calm, and specific, you can become just you. How refreshing.

You are the maker of your identity. You are your own universe. You re-create and design your own version of reality, which you then live in and project onto people, places, and things. Can you see that you have the power to create yourself anew? Will you embrace this power? Will you acknowledge this power? When will you assume responsibility? What good is your power if you don't use it?

It is time to rewrite your rulebook and determine your values. Observe and take charge of your own thoughts. Become your own master. If you are not your own master, who or what is? That's a pretty scary thought.

It is also time to address a formula for balance. The discussion and set of exercises that follow will inevitably spotlight behaviors, beliefs, and actions that lead to imbalance. Knowing what *not* to do is sometimes more helpful than knowing what to do. Engage the things that lead to your well-being and eliminate those that lead to your demise.

You need to author yourself. You need to invent yourself. You need to distinguish yourself. To enrich yourself. To invest yourself. To craft and sculpt yourself.

You have to do lots of work to change many things *within* yourself so that you can change many things *outside* yourself. If you want to change your external experience and circumstances, you need to change your internal experience.

Like a flower opening, this process of redefinition and redirection is truly not an event. It is a process. You must, therefore, expect small growth before the big blossoms appear in your life.

Beliefs and Values

Your beliefs, values, thoughts, and emotions become your self-designed architectural structure, which automatically perpetuates your decisions and impulsive actions. *You are your values and beliefs.* Unfortunately, many people never stop to question what they believe and value. They have unquestioningly taken on the values and beliefs of their parents or society with little or no personal thought. End of discussion.

Unfortunately, what ends up happening is exactly that. There is no discussion, no inner dialogue, no relationship with self. People who are unhappy with themselves find that they have not developed a relationship *with* self. Building a relationship with self requires some kind of internal dialogue. It is time to listen to your heart and become your own person.

If you always do what you've always done, you'll always get what you've always got and if nothing changes, nothing changes.

What do *you* value? Do you know?

Exercise

Identify fifty personal values. Please, do this now.

Separate the beliefs and values passed on to you from those that genuinely come from your heart. This may take time and will definitely require honesty and thoughtfulness. Now take the brainstorm list and, one by one, prioritize your fifty values, cutting and numbering one after another until you are left with only one top value. Calibrate your value system from one to fifty. What can you not live without? By doing this exercise, you will determine what you truly value and what you only care for. Expect this to be hard, but also expect it to be illuminating.

What makes a value important is that it is important to you. Perhaps you have found that you value honesty and integrity or fun and excitement. What do you do to align yourself with your values? What do you do that is incongruent with your values? This is not something you work at. This is something you *are*. A baby doesn't work at being accepted; she or he is accepted and valued for self.

Your spiritual identity, while here in this physical realm, is a composite of your values and beliefs—the driving force behind all that follows. Introduce your values to yourself, for your spiritual identity consists of these beliefs. Your spiritual view is self-determined through identification of your values and beliefs. Continue clarification of your values and beliefs in this lifetime. Take ownership of your spiritual identity. Know who you are so you can be who you are.

It all begins with values. Values generate thoughts. Thoughts generate emotions. Emotions generate attitudes. Attitudes generate actions and behaviors.

Observe Your Thoughts

Imagine a warm summer day. You are in a field of wildflowers. The breeze is softly waving the grasses around you. Fluffy clouds float in a sky of blue. You walk toward the sound of moving water while a sparrow chirps nearby and a frog jumps to the other side of the creek. You sit down on the edge of the water and relax.

Close your eyes and be there for a few minutes. What do you see? What do you hear? What do you think? What do you experience? Sink and soak in it.

Probably, you were able to visualize this scene and may even have added details to the calming atmosphere. Your thoughts may have reflected love, nature, or the possibilities before you. In contrast, had you been invited to imagine a horrible scene, your thoughts would probably reflect the negative aspects of that scene. Garbage in, garbage out.

Beauty in, beauty out.

You must think better before you feel better. Take charge of your thoughts. Direct your own thinking. This is the foundation to health. Your actions and behaviors will go where your head goes.

You can follow only what's in your head (your thoughts), so your actions go where your thinking goes. What do you choose to think about? What percentage of your thoughts are positive and functional? What percentage of your thoughts are negative and dysfunctional? What are you thinking now? Intentional thinking is the key, then mindfulness continues to monitor the process.

In working with your thoughts, you first need to intercept them. Try this after you put this book down today: When you are having any type of emotional response, *examine your thoughts.* Do they make sense? Are they true? Do they serve a productive function? Do they lead you in a positive direction? Do they produce a desired emotional response? Sort out positive from negative thoughts. Realize they are all just thoughts. You are their author. Take time to think about your thinking.

A positive thought is one that explains things and suggests how to change things if you choose to. Indecisive thoughts hinge on procrastination in choosing a direction. Solutions arise when you commit to a direction, yet retain the right to change your mind about anything at any time. After all, life is always in motion, and variables change. The tree reserves the right to change the direction in which its branches grow; nature demands intelligence for healthy survival. Don't be outdone by a tree.

Next, question the beliefs you inherited from your parents, relatives, teachers, peers, and society. Don't believe everything you were told, just believe the rational, helpful things, then sift through and throw out the irrational, hurtful things. Black-and-white thinking and all-or-nothing tendencies need to be revisited. The problem with black-and-white thinking is that reality is gray.

Give yourself permission to choose what you will and what you will not think and believe. These are *your* thoughts and *your* beliefs! In reading this book, take what we share here and decide what you will make your own. Give yourself permission to decide for yourself. It's all about employing your free will. Be true to yourself.

Too often, people say, "So-and-so made me mad/glad/afraid/sad." The truth of the matter is this: *You* made yourself mad/glad/afraid/sad. You are in control of your thoughts; therefore, you decide your response.

If someone tells you that you are worthless, you have two options: (A) Take the thought "I am worthless" and think it for yourself—thus experiencing the emotional response it gives you—or (B) think, "I am worthwhile" and experience the emotional response that thought gives you. What you choose to think is ultimately your decision. No one can make you think anything. At some level, you agree to the thought and make it your own.

As you rethink your beliefs and thoughts, take control of your emotional life. Your emotional control is directed by the brain's blindfolded functioning. This means that the human brain generates similar emotional feelings to imagined mental pictures as it does to similar real experiences. Witnessing a charging bear or picturing a charging bear provokes similar emotional responses. If you doubt this, observe someone watching a scary movie. If we think positive thoughts, we will experience positive results.

Otherwise, we become the victim and servant of our constricting mental constructs. Your thoughts and beliefs beget your feelings and consequent actions, so search your mind for positive power plants and channel your thoughts through them.

There's rarely any reason for you to feel bad unless you *choose* to or manufacture the event. Remember, your interpretations of facts, your thoughts, and your beliefs beget your emotional responses. To stop emotional hurt, take control of your emotions. You craft your own version of reality and live within your construct.

If you don't like the way you feel, then change your perspective. If you don't want to weed your garden, rename the weeds to flowers. Then smell the roses.

Formula for Balance

Once you begin to recognize your patterns and tendencies, you will need a map to redirect and replace negative thought patterns and behaviors with positive thought patterns and behaviors. The following simple formula will assist you in your journey:

To have a healthy relationship with yourself is to be in balance: spiritually, mentally, physically, and emotionally; in work and in play; with 50 percent inner-world focus and 50 percent outer-world focus; being 90 percent in the present, 5 percent in the past, and 5 percent in the future. Where are you? In balance or out of balance?

Like the universe, you, too, can come to perfect balance. As you do so, you contribute to a greater balance in this world, today and tomorrow.

In tribal ways, balance is health. Imbalance is disease. Health is the equilibrium between inward and outward energy. A disruption of this energy causes disease and illness. The ancient circle is the integration of the individual—the bringing together of self spiritually, physically, mentally, and emotionally. The healing includes the restoration of all you disowned due to shame-based criticism. Through implementing the formula of balance given above, you will come to recognize that you can become a self-determined and self-directed individual. To the proportion described above, be in the now, stay out of the head, and experience life. The farthest distance in the universe is from the head to the heart! We live life by experiencing life. We observe life with our mind. Heighten your senses so you can experience. You can't be spiritual in your head, only in your heart. You might have some nice thoughts in your head, but spirituality is an emotional connection and experience.

Take a complete and comprehensive inventory of your being and lifestyle now. What is it that you do or don't do on a daily basis? Look at all the components of the aforementioned formula and analyze where you are personally. Remember, balance is health. Sickness is imbalance.

Now strategize. Make a list of what you need to acquire spiritual, mental, physical, and emotional strength. Add work and play expectations into your weekly schedule to achieve balance. In other words, when will you physically exercise? Specifically, what days, what times? When will you spiritually exercise—pray, meditate, conduct or participate in ceremonies? Where and when? What mental exercises will you do? When will you read, learn, ponder? What mental food will you consume? Will this mental food nourish your mind or poison it with mental pollution? The rest of you will follow your head, so be careful what you put in it. How will you exercise your emotions? Ask yourself occasionally, "What am I feeling: mad, sad, glad, afraid, ashamed, hurt, frustrated?" and so on. What will you communicate to your loved ones? Do you hug? Can you touch another person? What music or artistic avenues do you give your emotions? Stimulate your endorphins, lift your spirits up, and transcend.

Make sure you leave plenty of time and room for fun and play. A life void of fun is an empty life at best. If you make life fun, you don't accumulate stress. If you don't make life fun, you need to find other ways to get stress out. Recently, one of Blackwolf's aged aunts died. She refused her medication and chose to die. When asked why she wanted to die, she said, "[Life's] no fun anymore." A wise woman she was. Don't be such a serious demanding tyrant or so carefree that there's no responsibility or accountability. There needs to be a balance.

You are not just a physical being, nor are you simply a spiritual being. You are also a mental and emotional being. You must respect all four *integrated* aspects of yourself just as Blackwolf's aunt did. Consciousness is collective in nature, for the whole is greater than the sum of the parts. Do your best to integrate all aspects of yourself. This requires balancing your time and attention in all four areas of your life. A life of integration and balance becomes the dawn for a new generation. What sunset experience will you offer the seventh generation? Our sunset is another's sunrise, so make your day beautiful.

You get only one body, and it becomes what you make of it. Are disease, obesity, and addictions obstructing your path to integration? There are only four things to consider: Balance, balance, balance, and balance!

Likewise, if you pray hard, but never play hard, you will be out of balance and suffer the consequences. If you learn, but do not love, you have neglected the very core of your identity. If you always cry, but never laugh, you have tipped the balancing wheel into dysfunction. In the same way, if you only laugh and cannot cry, you deny healing to your spirit. There are two types of tears, salty and sweet. Life is bittersweet. Nature demands this balance.

We are all extroverts and introverts to varying degrees. However, knowing our tendencies, we have an obligation to self to exercise the other. Work to be 50 percent inner- and 50 percent outer-world focused.

Do you truly live in the present? Or does your mind constantly plan, hope, and wish or regret, review, and complain? How much of the present do you really live? This formula asks you to be 90 percent here, now . . . and now . . . and now. . . . Practicing your listening awareness or mindfulness will help you in this endeavor. You will experience the benefits of this aspect of the formula immediately. Spend 5 percent of your time and attention in the past and 5 percent in the future. Respect the past; do not live there. Learn from your mistakes; honor what came before now and again, but in small doses. Create the future, but don't live there, either, for then you'll never live today.

Live the present. Live every moment. Don't worry about dying because you'll live every moment until you finally return to the spirit world. It's that simple.

Remember: *To have a healthy relationship with yourself is to be in balance: spiritually, mentally, physically, and emotionally; in work and in play; with 50 percent inner-world focus and 50 percent outer-world focus; being 90 percent in the present, 5 percent in the past, and 5 percent in the future.*

Becoming more and more conscious of this formula and implementing its principles will grant you a more balanced life, thus a more harmonious relationship with yourself.

Become your potential. Only then can you experience the secret of life, which is simply to live life and experience the experience.

One Step at a Time

Hiking the Greenstone Trail, the thirty-five-mile backbone of Isle Royale in Lake Superior, is a lesson in *moments*. One does not begin the hike—carrying forty pounds of gear, managing difficult topography—with the notion to get to the other end of the island *now*. Obviously, the hiker realizes that the trail will demand much more from him or her than simply thinking about the hike, planning the course of crossing contour lines over the kitchen table, and imagining the end result. However necessary this planning and visualization is, it will not get you to the other end. Only *you* can get yourself to the other end of the island, one step at a time. Inch by inch, it's a cinch. So goes your life, moment by moment. It is not magic.

Coming into a functional, healthy relationship with yourself also is achieved one step at a time. The path that you are on will require planning, but as with all successful achievements, it is in the *doing* that ideas are realized.

Many challenges parallel the journey you are now on, in many ways. *First, your strength will be tested.* The journey you are choosing may be hard at times. In the process of becoming, you will experience times you think you can't endure, but you will. You will become stronger. Each step strengthens us and begins to eliminate our weaknesses. Many steps are easily recognizable. One step requires trust.

Second, know that difficulties are up ahead. Take a moment to anticipate some of the challenges you may face as you begin working on your formula of balance. What roadblocks will you encounter? How will you make your way around them? Who will discourage you? Why? How will you respond? What will you do or not do to sabotage your own growth? Write down the answers to these questions. Anticipate other difficulties. Please, do this now.

There will be times when the challenges you face appear to be insurmountable. Seek within yourself the determination to find a way around the difficulty. Recognize that you cannot anticipate all of the difficulties to come. Call on your spiritual reserve. You are capable of so much! If you can picture it, you can probably do it. Visualize to vitalize.

Third, your growth may be painful. Pain, for everyone, is a great part of life and should not always be avoided. Pain is any unpleasant physical or emotional sensation. Pain is a normal, useful part of life and may warn of trouble. Physical pain may tell us we are injured or weak. Emotional pain tells us there is something wrong in our experience.

Western culture has a tendency to avoid pain, to subdue it with medication or minimize the emotional response to it. The only healthy way to deal with our emotional pain is to acknowledge it and identify it, verbally, within a trusting, intimate relationship. Physical pain also needs to be acknowledged and endured in order to raise our pain threshold. We can learn to manage our pain the same way we can learn to manage our thoughts and emotions. Pain can become a doorway to self-discipline and another way to experience self. Don't fear pain. Write your own life rules. Be responsible. It leads to freedom and the ability to accept yourself. Be true to yourself.

Like an athlete whose body expels toxins, you, too, will expel your toxins, cleansing yourself of the things that weigh you down and poison your system. We dread the discomfort or pain that accompanies growth. You need to realize that this is okay. Implementing the formula for balance will require discipline and may indeed be painful. Become aware of your own presence. Turn your pain into power. Power is like the gasoline in your fuel tank.

In addition, you may need to expel toxic emotions such as anger, resentment, guilt, remorse, and shame, which block you from embracing the sacredness of all. You will be healthier because of it. These poisons block you from experiencing your own body's and mind's natural healing rhythms.

To do this, you need to identify these emotions and not deny or dilute them. What anger, resentment (relived anger), guilt, remorse (relived guilt), or shame do you harbor? Notice that anger and resentment are projected outside of us—externally focused—while guilt, shame, and remorse are within us. Take time now to identify your toxins. What do you harbor? What were the circumstances? Who are you angry with? Why? Do you direct anger inside or outside you? Be as specific in your response as you can be. Who is your lightning rod? Yourself or others?

Do you beat yourself up with internal dialogue? Do you value or devalue yourself?

Now look at the toxins you wrote down. Experience each one. Verbalize them with another human being who can empathize and validate what you are feeling. Get it out. Talk about it. Feel it. Experience it. These energies are only destructive when they are ignored. So, talk to your anger. Talk to your grief. Talk to your fear and regard these emotions as if they were people. Ask them what they want you to do, what they want you to understand, and what they want you to give attention to. Listen with a sharp ear and you will hear. Trust. Write down what your emotions are telling you. Within this dialogue, you will find yourself. Find yourself to be yourself.

Once you have accomplished these steps, you need to accept your humanity. Recognize that you are a human being. Humans make mistakes. That is life. You are here to experience life. If you're not perfect, then you are perfectly adequate. Don't be afraid of making mistakes because that's how we learn. Life is a learning process, and by the time we begin to figure it out, it's time to go back home to the spirit world. The only thing we will ever do perfectly is die. Don't worry. You won't screw it up. Take this time now to forgive yourself and others. Please, do this now. Verbally forgive. Forgiveness removes the thorn from the foot.

Now you are ready to convert this exercise into a learning experience for similar future challenges. Having discharged the physical energy of the emotion, the mental content can now evaporate.

Finally, you must exercise your flexibility. Without this, you are doomed to fail. As with any new exercise, we may resist stretching at first, yet without this step our tightened muscles will force us to stop. Do not sabotage your journey before you begin. Stretch your spiritual, mental, physical, and emotional muscles carefully and patiently. Slow down your steps; the end of the trail will be there. Make sure you will be there, too.

What keeps one on the path of change will be the knowledge and trust that all the effort will pay off in the end. A new, fit body, mind, spirit, and emotional being will emerge from the fire. You are being purified as gold by fire. Yield to the process; it is a process, after all, and not an event.

Learn the steps to becoming who are you: visualize, verbalize, and vitalize. First, be conscious of your values and beliefs. That is who you are. Visualize what you want to become. Picture it. Verbalize the changes you need to make. Say it. Finally, vitalize. Do it. Become it.

The following four tips will help you maintain the course:

1. Recognize that you are not alone. Others who are serious about realizing their potential are going through the exact same thing. This will bring you some comfort and strength. Find others who are following a path of personal growth. Stick with them.

2. Believe in yourself. Tap your internal trust and feed yourself messages of encouragement. Know that the path you chose is the path you chose. Consistently remind yourself of the rewards and the reasons you took this path originally. Commend yourself on each tiny success. Look in the mirror and say, "You're becoming! I see a change!" Develop your own mantra and repeat it often throughout the day: *I am working on* _____. Add a picture to go with your verbalization. What will you visualize? By verbalizing and visualizing your message to yourself, you will be strengthening your resolve and reminding yourself of what is important to you. Consider doing this at least once an hour. Then you may reduce this to five times a day. Decide which one thing you will focus on for that day.

3. Begin today with a plan. Determine where it is you want to go and how you will get there. Truly, *those who fail to plan, plan to fail.* Ask yourself what you want to gather from this lifetime and what you want to contribute in your lifetime. What brings you joy? That is your direction. Set your goals. Make a plan. And remember that if you always do what you've always done, you'll always get what you always got. If nothing changes, then nothing changes. Decide carefully what it is you want to do or become. Be specific. Make it measurable, if possible. For example: *I will eat healthy foods today. I will say two encouraging messages to those I love today. I will take an hour walk in order to connect to my inner self and exercise my body. I will notice three positive qualities about the person I am having difficulty loving or liking.* Be sure to implement the formula for balance in your planning. But do not overplan; be flexible in your daily decisions. Reserve the right to change your mind about anything at any time. Stay the course, but do not *become* the course. Leave room for intuition and trust your instincts.

4. Share your progress with another. This is vital. Have someone you can talk to about what is difficult and what growth you already notice. This person may be a colleague, counselor, or best friend. Find someone whom you can trust to talk about your progress. Who in your life would listen without judgment?

Celebrate! Celebrate all that you are becoming. Celebrate just being! Celebrate the new you! Celebrate this moment, now! Take time to massage your being with the touch that only you can give yourself. What can you do for yourself that would really be nice? Time alone? A walk? Your favorite music? Dancing? A relaxing bath? Honor yourself. Compliment yourself. Take care of yourself. If you don't, who will? Write yourself a note. What does it say? Need to change something in your life? Do it.

Perhaps the greatest advice ever given came in six words: *Inch by inch, it's a cinch!* Remind yourself of this adage and you, too, will complete the challenging course of coming home to yourself. In the celebration of self, a celebration for others will begin to emerge. Take a victory lap and see how good it feels.

Chapter Five

Celebrate You

The ultimate experience of life is death. Have you ever thought about your own funeral? Who would be there? What would they say? How would others be affected? How would you be honored? Thinking about one's own funeral is not necessarily a symptom of necrophilia. As you live your life, you must consider the end at some point and become aware of your own mortality. As you glimpse into the future, come nearer the door of the next generations. When your door closes, another opens.

Have you ever been recognized or honored, other than at your birth or subsequent birthdays, for who you are, not what you've done? How many people ever receive such a tremendous gift? What would you like to hear at your own funeral?

Take this opportunity to go to your own funeral. Picture the flowers. See your loved ones. Listen to the words and music. What do you notice? Look around the room. See the people standing and sitting, talking and remembering. Who is there? What are they saying about you? Are their words filled with vague tributes? Do you hear specific words of honor? In what ways did you contribute? What legacy did you leave? Now hear the silence. It says more than words. How do these people feel about you? We invite you to write this down now.

Eventually, notice there is one person standing to the side of all this activity. Go up to that person and ask why she or he thinks you are such a special person to be honored. Ask this person how she or he knew you. Then turn this person around and notice this person is you.

All that you have done will no longer matter. All that you collected will not matter. Awards and accomplishments will no longer matter. Do you know what will matter to this person standing to the side of your coffin? What will this person say about you? What attention, affection, recognition, and approval will *you* have to give to *yourself?* Ultimately, only you can answer.

Take time now to write out this scenario.

All people need attention, affection, recognition, and approval. Many relationships begin with this exchange and continue to validate one another out of love.

For some, however, this need becomes a bottomless pit, especially if it were never adequately met in childhood. Most people look outside themselves for self-esteem via these four basic needs of attention, affection, recognition, and approval. Looking from person to person, status symbol to status symbol, they try in vain to get from outside themselves what can only come from within. That is why self-esteem is called *self*-esteem rather than *other*-esteem: It must come from within self. Come to realize you cannot take any of these external approvals with you on your final journey. You will take only yourself, your thoughts, your experiences, your spirit. Who do you want to be? How do you want to meet this day? Who are you truly? How will you celebrate yourself?

It is time now to consider your very existence. You! Not what you do, not what you have accomplished. Not what you have. Not even how others respond to you. Just *you!*

Celebrate you. Give yourself the attention, affection, recognition, and approval you deserve. Play and have fun in life. Enjoy who you are! Honor yourself with deliberate attention. Love yourself, appreciate your uniqueness, and participate in life in a way that makes you and others more, rather than less. This is the yeast for growing healthy generations to come.

Loving Your Being

Do you love your being?

Recall the first reflection exercise of this book. Once more, we would like you to evaluate yourself. Right now, on a scale from one to ten, determine once more how you feel about yourself (one being self-rejection, ten being fully content with self). How do you feel about yourself? Do you like yourself? Tolerate yourself? Love yourself? Hate yourself? Are you in good company when you are alone? Has this number changed as you have come to know yourself better?

If you answered anything other than a ten, you are in need of a very simple tenet that builds harmonious relationships: *Add value, rather than devalue.* The lower the number, the more you need to add value to self. This is critical in dealing with your relationship with yourself. All other relationships depend on how healthy a relationship you have with yourself. You cannot give what you do not have.

More than likely, growing up in the abusive system you probably did, you are very familiar with some of the infinite ways people devalue self or others. Emotional and verbal abuses are more commonplace than we, as a society, would like to admit. Name-calling, belittling, shaming, and sabotaging are just some ways we hurt others and ourselves. What have you said to yourself today that belittled your spirit? In what ways were you disappointed with self? How do you sabotage your personal growth? What part of you would you rather disown? Have you beaten yourself up verbally today?

Whatever the cause for crippling self-rejection or hatred, we end up being our own therapists and can arrive at our own resolutions. You must add your own value! You must reconstruct self rather than destruct self. If you don't, who will?

Loving your being is evidenced through self-validation and self-endorsement. It is up to you to give yourself the attention, affection, recognition, and approval that you need. The source is within. Put your ego in your back pocket. Your ego is full of fear and needs an inordinate amount of attention, affection, recognition, and approval. *It is not about doing and getting. It is about being and giving.* Your spirit is a self-validating, fearless being. Come to your basic nature and soak in your own presence.

Accept yourself for who you really are, both male and female, logical and emotional, light side and dark side, physical and mental—all integrated energy.

Integration is paramount because every unloved slice of our personality will become hostile. The tyrant within is fueled and energized by self-rejection. Perhaps the greatest tragedy in the universe is self-rejection. Self-rejection diminishes our worth to an abyss of fear and rage, spewing aggression and abandonment.

Remember, you were born a global fire of self-love. No wonder humans have instinctual urges to return to the womb, wherein lie memories of unconditional love and total acceptance. As newborns, we were yet in harmony with the universe. We must communicate to ourselves self-validation and self-endorsement. It cannot come from anyone else.

Go back to the beginning, when you were simply you. Be born again. In your rebirth, give yourself the love no one else can. Take this time, now, to accept and honor all that you are.

Talk first to your body. Thank your body for all that it does for you. Go through each body part and validate its contribution. Thank your feet for carrying you all these years. Honor your legs for their strength and stamina. Recognize all the work your hands have done: tying your shoelaces, feeding you, washing you, writing, and lifting. Attend to even the scars on your skin, the aches in your muscles. Thank them for their protection and messages. Thank all of you for being you. Give love to your physical body.

Now communicate with your mind. Listen to what your mind tells you. Thank your mind for its energy and direction. Accept the light and the dark sides, realizing one complements the other. See thoughts as thoughts, no more, no less. Accept your human nature. Know your mind is more than your thoughts. Honor its mystery. When Blackwolf presented a fifty-year sobriety medallion to a very close Mohican friend, his elder's comment was, "It's hard to imagine the deep significance of this mystery."

Recognize the knowledge your mind has gained. Marvel in the understandings you have made your own. Attend to the thoughts. Attend to the silence between the thoughts. Extend love to your mind.

Communicate next with your emotions. Don't be afraid of your emotions. They are awareness energy and need to be experienced. They tell you what your mind cannot tell you. Listen to the pain and pleasure. Honor both your gentleness and courage; experience both the male and female aspects of yourself. See your emotions as messengers. They are leading you to future growth. Pain is a powerful teacher. Acknowledge and grieve for all that you have lost. Be with your emotions—the anger, the happiness, the sadness, the fear, the excitement, the grief. Respect your emotions, and they will respect you.

Now, connect with your spirit. Touch the timeless aspect of who you are. Feel the vibrations within. Hum and vibrate your spiritual being for comfort. Pause in silence. Slow down to experience the spiritual awakening that is for all people. Attend. Be mindful. Be.

Love your spirit. Thank your spirit. Feel your spirit pulsate.

Come to self in order to be self, in order to experience self, in order to celebrate self, in order to enjoy self, in order to expand self and fulfill self.

Appreciate Your Uniqueness

What color are you?

If you could choose just one color to represent you, what would it be? Why? What does that color do for you? How does it make you feel? What images come to mind? What temperature? What emotions? Your answers to these questions will mirror who you are. This is the color of your spirit. Isn't it grand to see yourself in this way?

Knowing your uniqueness will help you find your niche in the universe. As you come to celebrate who you are, you celebrate the past, present, and future.

The tribal way to find your personal reflection is to see yourself in nature. Ask yourself what animal, bird, element, or spirit you are like in nature. The combination of these attributes and affinities will illuminate your essence.

Now consider what you chose. Write down all the characteristics you can think of that this aspect of nature possesses. What do you discover? Find the parallels in your life. Notice how you are reflected in that animal, bird, or element. What attributes of that animal, fish, bird, tree, or flower do you have an affinity with? Acclaim all that you are! Celebrate this discovery. Find yourself in nature to fulfill your natural niche.

You are unique because of your difference, not your sameness. Go outside and pick out a blade of grass. Just one blade of grass. Look at it. Notice how it is different from those next to it. Realize that there are no two blades of grass exactly alike. Realize that there is no one like you. Celebrate your uniqueness.

How are you special? What did the Creator bestow upon you that makes you uniquely you? Celebrate that knowledge and difference! What special wood do you bring to the fire of life?

You open and close somewhat like a flower, and you never open or close your personality and character exactly in the same way. You and all of creation are constantly in flux and change. Celebrate your uniqueness. Celebrate your changing hues.

Notice how you enjoy being around others who like themselves, who are happy and excited with life. As they celebrate themselves, they celebrate all that supports their existence. In this celebration, the seventh generation also benefits. It cannot not benefit. Honoring promotes honoring. Adding value promotes more value. To honor all of creation is to honor yourself simultaneously, as you are also a necessary and integral part of the web of life and future generations.

Find an artistic way to express your uniqueness. Design your own symbol, one that best represents who you are. Write a poem. Sing a song. Dance. Sculpt something that will carry you beyond the physical realm. Color. Press your hand in wet cement. Artists and poets are in quiet connection with their spirit and the eternal source of all of creation. Allow the creator to move through you. Create!

Every person's spirit is a universe in and of itself. Within you is a universe of possibilities to explore and celebrate. Travel inward to new frontiers. Witness the spiraling of internal galaxies as you discover your likes and dislikes. Know who you are, and then discover more of you. It is never-ending. Your self-discovery will go on for infinity. The excitement of learning about yourself will never end. Take this time to finish the statements that follow. In the form of a poem, you will verbalize and celebrate who you are.

I Am

I wonder _____

I feel _____

I see _____

I want _____

I love _____

I try _____

I smile _____

I am _____

I worry _____

I cry _____

I pretend _____

I touch _____

I struggle _____

I hear _____

I dream _____

I am _____

I understand _____

I say _____

I know _____

I discover _____

I honor _____

I hope _____

I pray _____

I am _____

Work to Live, not Live to Work

You, you, and you.

Sometimes it's good to be self-reliant. If you are self-reliant about your health, you will be sure to take good care of yourself. It is also good to consider yourself special, because you are. Declare your birthday a holiday!

Work may well be your demon in disguise. You probably were conditioned to value or devalue yourself relative to your reluctance or investment in work. In many cases, the worker becomes the servant rather than the master. All too often, in this culture, work controls the person and self-esteem is confused with work-esteem. Again, self-esteem is called self-esteem because it needs to come from self. If not, it would have been called work-esteem or something else.

What is work? Most people would limit this to mean our jobs, how we earn our livings. Many people are more interested in a paycheck than a profession. It is great to have a skill, trade, or profession that will adequately provide for your basic economic needs. But what if your work was also your play? Everyone can play at work. Whatever your job, there are always appropriate opportunities to be playful. Don't be so serious! Remember, work to live, don't live to work. Realize that your job is meant to assist your living. Your living is not to revolve around your work.

Take this time to consider your relationship with your work. Is it healthy? Does it demand a disproportionate amount of your free time? Do you take your job home? Do you get your esteem from what you do, rather than who you are? What exactly is your relationship with your job? When you die, will you wish you had spent more time at the office?

Now let's go further. *Work* is defined as any physical or mental energy directed to the accomplishment of something.

This definition goes beyond your job to all that you do that involves your energy. This more inclusive definition may give you further insight into how and what you value. How do you spend your energy to accomplish a healthy relationship with yourself? Consider your daily activities outside the job atmosphere. How do you spend your energy? Positively or negatively?

Write these activities down. Is your energy expended in ways that reduce stress or add stress? Do you work for yourself, or do you work for the expectations of others? For example, do you cut your grass to live up to the expectations of your neighbor, or do you cut the grass because it simultaneously gives you pleasure and physical exercise? There is a big difference. One alleviates stress. Another promotes further stress. Live life by your rules; it's *your* life. Be true to yourself. This is probably the greatest rule of all.

There are many ways you can spend your energy to help develop a healthy personal relationship and reduce stress. Think back on the last two days. Have you done something fun? Have you given and received touch and affection? Did you do one thing at a time? Have you overloaded? Did you get frequent exercise? Did you stretch? Did you drink plenty of water and juices? Were you mindful? Have you played?

Have you been able to get rid of stress? Four of the best ways to reduce physical stress are shaking, having an orgasm, crying, and laughing. Of course, some are more appropriate given certain circumstances, but they are all valid, nonetheless. Be open to reducing stress. Realize that laughing is indeed good medicine. Crying is not just for women. Allow yourself the right to experience your nature.

Consider the following to assist the energy you emit: Eat at least one balanced meal per day, get plenty of sleep, be appropriate weight for your height, organize your time effectively, talk openly about domestic issues, define your spiritual values, smile, take daily quiet time, and have your personal spot, a place you can retreat to for rejuvenation. Everyone has a personal spot on Mother Earth's lap. Where is yours?

Enjoy!

Perhaps one of the first things the Creator will ask you upon your return home to the spirit world will be, "Did you enjoy?"

"Did you enjoy the birds I gave you, the beauty I made? Did you enjoy the people I placed in your life? Did you enjoy the strawberry in June? Did you enjoy the music and the rhythms? Did you enjoy the seasons, the colors, the depths, the heights? Did you enjoy the sunrise and sunset? Did you enjoy the water, the snow, the rain, the sun, the moon? Did you enjoy your passions? Did you enjoy other people's passions? Did you enjoy aging? Did you enjoy the laughter? Did you enjoy the children? Did you enjoy moving your body, walking, skipping, running, swimming, dancing? Did you enjoy creating? Did you enjoy art? Did you enjoy warm fires and cool shade? Did you enjoy a good joke? Did you enjoy the evenings and the mornings? Did you enjoy playing? Did you enjoy the animals, the insects, the plants, the still ones? Did you enjoy each breath? Did you enjoy being you? Did you enjoy the experience of living and of being you?"

Do you enjoy? Do you enjoy being you? If you truly enjoy your own company, you can never be lonely. How do you enjoy yourself? What lifts your spirit? What makes you carefree? How does your spirit experience freedom? Whatever gives you joy, that is your direction.

People really need to follow their heart, their bliss. If you can't enjoy life, what is the point? Even Viktor Frankl, in a Nazi concentration camp, was able to enjoy the sunset. Enjoyment is only limited by you.

Take this time to write down the things you truly enjoy. Create a list for you to go back to for your own enjoyment. You deserve to enjoy! In fact, enjoyment may be a spiritual expectation. Joy is of the spirit world, so transcend the visible and embrace the invisible to touch the mysteries of life and the secrets of creation.

Break free from the false beliefs that entrap and imprison you. Fill that new void with joy and the excitement of being a freed spirit. Once you have experienced this freedom, you can never be the same. You will care less about consequences, and your enjoyment is contagious. People like to be around people who enjoy life. The Creator probably does, too. Does this seem too simple? Please don't trip on simplicity.

Extend!

We are all going down the river of life, and the world is here to support us on our journeys.

You will make your life journey, as all people of all time make theirs. Yet, no two life journeys will be exactly alike. You must take your journey alone, for your journey is an internal event. Your parents, teachers, and life experiences gave you the maps and the compass to carry. Now you have the opportunity to fashion from that your own path. Your journey will become a series of choices, and you will live with the consequences of those choices, positive or negative. You are the author of your life event. It is time to be accountable to yourself. Begin anew.

Assert your rights. You have rights to privacy; to information; to ask for what you need and what you want; to express your feelings and opinions; to say no and not feel guilty, shameful, or selfish; to make your own choices; to make lifestyle changes; to decide who will and will not touch you; to make mistakes and learn from them; to be interdependent; to know who has accused you of something; to set limits and boundaries; to feel good about yourself; to think about your thinking and change it; to have fun and author your life story.

In the darkness of your spirit is a labyrinth of choices, fears, and hopes, yet when you come to see with spiritual eyes that require no direction, when you trust the innermost part of your being, you are free to fly above the dead ends, the frustrations, the imaginings of your mind. You will intuitively gravitate to the one direction of your spirit. Like the birds that fly south for the winter, your spirit knows which way is home. It is beyond thinking. In today's world, it is risky business to assert the power of intuition. Yet to those of you who are truly moving with the currents of the spirit world, the results speak of authenticity. Congruency grows out from the insights and the knowing that emerge from one in contact with his or her spiritual power and birthright. In like manner, people who listen to their inner silence recognize the need to be here, now.

Too often, so-called spiritual journeys take ardent followers into a maze. But those who see with clouded eyes become lost in dead ends and myriad directions. They may become obsessed with powerful promises, unable to see the greater view that will show them the possibilities in life. They may be unable or unwilling to live here (on earth) now, to be fully alive, functioning, and contributing to the one great family. Cults and religious fanatics sadly remind us of the destructive force that emerges from such spiritual starvation. This is precisely why you must first focus on your relationship with yourself. When that focus is clear, you will be best prepared to decide for yourself what you value and believe. Do the inward work now, and you will not be distracted with outward appearances and people pleasing. Fulfill your own expectations. Ultimately, you answer only to yourself and your Creator.

Do you wear your spirituality with loud colors, jangling with too many bangles? Or, in contrast, do you wear the simple clothes of silence and look up with a peaceful, clear countenance? These are the people who have listened well, who experience bliss and who honor all as they honor themselves. These are the few who do not claim to have the answers to life's most profound questions, for they accept the mystery in every mystery. They may say nothing, but in doing so, they say it all.

These are people who are easily recognized by our spirits. We instantly feel comfortable within their presence. We immediately let out a long-awaited breath of release. We understand and are understood. We are more when we are with them. They do not take, do not push, do not pretend, do not judge, do not point. They just are. Notice how their presence affects your presence today and tomorrow. Keep this tenet in mind, for just as this is true for others, it is also true for you.

Your path is of extreme importance, a source of life for you and others who are in need of your guidance, support, energy, touch, love, and validation. Your path may provide love and healing for others who walk beside you, even if just for the year, month, week, day, hour, or minute. Your influence by your example is unfathomable.

Eyes look to see sacred mountains. Ears hear the rivers of life. Look and listen within. This is where it all begins and ends.

When you see yourself not merely as a physical body but as spirit, what have you to fear? If you see the world as an extension of your physical and spiritual self, then you can care about all things. Then you can respect all.

As you continue to identify who you are, redirect and redesign your life energies. As you come to celebrate your life, you are positioned to become one of those people who quietly, yet profoundly, affect the world today and tomorrow. Develop and maintain a healthy relationship with yourself. By doing so, the ripples in the water will become contagious inspirations to others. The seventh generation will experience your growth. May your life help all who will come to enter a healthier world than you did. May you leave the world better than you found it.

Remember, *we,* not *me!*

PART THREE

UNDERSTANDING
YOUR
RELATIONSHIPS

Chapter Six

Healthy Balance

It doesn't take a baby long before he or she realizes that life includes a lot more than self. Indeed, we are all aware of the separation anxiety that children experience as they consider life separate from their mothers. Healthy children, nonetheless, grow with the ability to maintain separateness, yet honor those with whom they walk.

Living and loving while always mindful of others is definitely an art. For example, in an unhealthy, enmeshed family system, some members may blur the line between themselves and others, so that instead of a sense of *we,* narcissism dominates. Others may separate to the point of total disregard of others, and dysfunction and aloofness result. Few in today's world truly live and love and learn the importance of individual autonomy complemented with a vision of the interrelatedness of all beings. Few experience a sense of being one within each other.

To live, love, and learn for the seventh generation, we not only look out for self, but for the six generations to follow. This vision for all seven generations is one of *we,* not *me.*

The best of visions, however, crumbles without the bond of love. Love is the glue.

Love gives you both the courage and freedom to look fearlessly at one's inevitable death without regret. For to know that you are complete in the experience of love is truly like having your heart overflow. As if it were a bucket, fill *your* heart to spill over with love. It is your heart to fill. It is *your* heart to spill. You haven't lived until you've loved.

We have an instinctual need to love and form relationships. We need others. However, we tend to complicate our relationships with the hierarchical and abusive residuals of the system in which we were raised. Our instinctual need to form relationships and to love is accompanied by our learned behavior and beliefs. The goal of Part Three is to distinguish the purity of instinct from dysfunctional tendencies.

You do not walk life's path alone. You encounter many people, places, and things along your journey and form relationships with them all in some way. Some relationships are intimate, some casual, and most merely coincidental. Although in your inner world you are always alone, in your outside world you are *never* alone. From momentary relationships to those of immeasurable depth, all relationships have the potential to fill our hearts, bring us closer to our spiritual essences, and prepare us for our glorious return home. What we fill up with here, we may well pour out there. What will be the contents of your heart? What treasures will you share with your Creator? What sacred truths will you bring back home to the spirit world once your life is over? What will you gather and share? Come to see that relationships with others are sacred. Be careful and deliberate about what you put in your bucket; it has an eternal fragrance.

Part Three will continue to address the balance that is required for all healthy relationships, guiding the new you to recognize and understand what healthy, balanced relationships with others are like. Your personal predispositions will be confronted. You will be helped to understand and extinguish patterns that interfere with truly healthy relationships, and, at the same time, be taught to integrate your personal formula for balance.

Necessary work is required of you if you are to become truly able to appreciate the precepts in the following chapters.

Love and loss will be discussed. The circle of love and the cycle of life will be honored. Here, you will reflect on your sacred role in relationships with others, in the loop of love. You will practice letting go. Some people equate letting go with losing. Remember, winning is a control issue. Letting go is non-control. Letting go will set you free. Eagle soars freely because his wingtips yield to volatile air currents, somewhat like shock absorbers. Eagle maintains control by letting go of control. The paradox is freeing.

Open your heart's floodgates. Allow all those with whom you share your day to rush into your heart. The possibilities of further fulfillment exist. Learn how to navigate between rough tides and negative forces that we all experience. Soar like Eagle.

Please do not allow your fears of rejection to stifle your attempts to establish intimate, meaningful, functional relationships. We always risk rejection within relationships. You won't die or go crazy if you are rejected. You may become hurt and sad, but those emotions will eventually evaporate, as all emotions do. You may also learn something of yourself and something of the other. There is no total loss in any relationship. There are no guaranteed relationships, only opportunities for growth—growth for all concerned because relationships are of mutual benefit. When those benefits are actualized, the relationship may terminate itself, as a branch may fall from the tree to make way for new growth.

Please do not allow your fears of connection to stifle your attempts at establishing intimate, meaningful, functional relationships, either. We also risk being known within functional relationships. You won't die or go crazy if someone can see your spirit. Instead, you may experience love and fulfillment. You may also learn something of yourself and something of the other. There is always something to gain as you come into relationship with another. A true friend accepts you as you are, with all your strengths and weaknesses. What you see is what you get.

We are not alone. We share the same breath, the same sky, the same time and space. As your breath recycles into the sky of the seventh generation, come to see that, indeed, we are present beyond our death. Where was the air that is in your lungs this moment four months ago? Was it in a panda in China? A zebra in Africa? A polar bear? Or a penguin? We all share the same breath. The circle continues. The seventh generation continues as you relate to those in your life. We are all related.

Picture this scene: A plane lifts off the runway of the Phoenix airport. Inside, a woman cradles an infant in her arms and soothes the child by swaying her body. The child coos, oblivious to what goes on beyond the security of her mother's arms. The baby's inner and outer worlds are in harmony. Satisfied, she gurgles, and her vocalization seems to soften the roar of the jet engine's thrust. The plane and its passengers cruise at thirty thousand feet while the baby remains in the sanctuary of her mother's arms. A sacred relationship on earth endures beyond sky.

Truly, this baby teaches lessons of balance and acceptance. Balanced internally and externally, she is present with the moment and what is inside her realm of influence. At birth, our inner world and outer world are equal. Our outer self reflects our inner experience. Accepting what is, there is no need to change or control the circumstance, nor is there fear of potential harm. The present moment and all it offers is all the infant knows. Her relationship with her mother is one of unconditional love, one for the other. Needs are expressed; needs are met. We could learn a lot from this mother/child relationship.

We must learn the same lessons of balance and acceptance about others in our life. Too often, we get caught up in the game of control, wanting to be writers, actors, and audience members all at once. Controlling behaviors upset balance, and an equal relationship cannot exist. When you think about it, what can you really control in your outside world, anyway?

Acceptance is compromised when we judge and become too narrow-minded to forgive. Too often, we believe that our perception is *the* perception, that our version of reality is the only one. Those who do not see life with our lenses become wrong. How can we accept that which we do not even acknowledge? How can we completely accept ourselves if we will not accept the diversity of others? Others mirror the changes in beliefs and values that we must go through if we are to arrive at our destiny. To judge is to be judged. Acknowledging only *one way* does not expand life views nor honor the mystery of life. Acknowledging many ways honors change and differences. Ever-new relationships can burgeon from such a point of departure. Different angles of perception illuminate the whole. Truly, none are so blind as those who will not see.

Indeed, relationships with others will assist you in finding out how you are doing in your relationship with yourself. A person who has mastered the premises of self, who is in balance spiritually, mentally, physically, and emotionally; in work and in play; with 50 percent inner-world focus and 50 percent outer-world focus; being 90 percent in the present, 5 percent in the past, and 5 percent in the future, has worked to balance his or her inner and outer worlds. Such a person understands the honesty, open-mindedness, patience, acceptance, and tolerance that are needed to develop a relationship with self and is able to apply these same qualities in a relationship with another.

Do you know what a healthy balance between two people looks like? Feels like? Sounds like? This chapter will lead you to discover how well you interact with others and whether you are helping or hurting the people in your lives, including yourself. What predispositions do you bring to each of your relationships? What patterns interfere with healthy interactions? What aspects of your personal formula must you implement to assist collaborative balance? You need to know what you want, otherwise all roads will lead you nowhere. Necessary work is to be done. Prepare to change. Prepare to make a difference with the seventh generation as you change your thinking and understanding in your relationships with others. You must first think better before you (and consequently, others) can feel better. Ultimately, you go where your head goes.

It is time to define, understand, and enhance your relationship with others. Acknowledge habitual tendencies and roles that interfere with sacred connections. Reflect upon your own expectations, honor interdependence, and assertively live and let live. This will provide nourishment for the next generations. Your commitment to growth, even if you struggle, will be felt sevenfold. You help others as you help yourself.

Victims of Our Own Expectations

Perhaps the biggest pitfall to be aware of when developing relationships with others is your own expectations. You truly can become the victim of your own expectations. What you expect of yourself and what you expect of others may interfere enormously with the dance of life.

What *do* you expect from yourself as you relate to other people? What is your role when you interact with others? Are you the mediator? The boss? The victim? The teacher? The jokester? The healer? Can you see that a role is not necessary when you are *developing* personal relationships? Obviously, we all assume certain roles in specific situations, as deemed necessary. Nevertheless, the best teachers, judges, bosses, and healers are those who are first themselves, then allow their roles to assist the exchange. The role (or job description) may serve a purpose at a given time, but, all too often, it interferes with the development of meaningful enduring relationships. Those who *become* the role have sacrificed themselves in the process. You are not your role! A role is simply a hat to wear to distinguish the circumstance. The chief executive officer of a major corporation may well take out the kitchen garbage when she or he gets home after work.

A teacher who is human first will always gain the respect of his or her students. A boss who relates to individuals and their needs will always be one people want to work with. A comedian who is caring first will always tickle an audience without threat. Actually, risky as it may sound, all that is needed in this world is you—without roles, just you.

It is important to realize that you are the same person in different roles, at different times, in different places, with different people. Do not confuse your personality and role with your being. Although your roles vary, your being is unchangeable.

Roles also tend to be judged. One may be seen as better than another. One seems more educated, more caring, more respected, and more powerful. This judging leads to a hierarchy in life. Thus, status symbols result.

Do you see yourself as inferior or superior in relationship to others? This is a vital question, as it may clarify a role you have taken on with others. Do you feel as comfortable chatting with a CEO, a doctor, or a millionaire as you do speaking with a salesclerk or a child? Do you feel as comfortable chatting with a salesclerk or a child as you do speaking with a physicist, an artist, or a priest?

Are you on equal footing with others or do you hesitate with some people, seeing yourself as less or more than them in some way? Too often, those who feel inferior and see others as superior take on the victim role. As you age, you may be like a vacuum sucking up negativism. You need to empty your dust bag. Develop yourself! Shed the victim role and empower yourself. You can only be as much as you give yourself the credit, power, and wisdom to be: inferior, superior, or equal. You set your own limits. You alone determine your level of self-esteem.

Likewise, those who feel superior and see others as inferior take on the abusive role. As you age, you may again be like the dust bag, this time exploding with its contents. Develop yourself! Shed the abusive role you learned and empower yourself with reflective truths. You have only as much compassion and wisdom as you give yourself. You can open your world to others.

Certainly, there are jobs and roles that require more education and more responsibility than others. Choices to participate in varying roles are simply choices. They are not the person. You are not your role. Remember that we all are waves of the same ocean. Sometimes we are little waves; sometimes we are big waves. There will always be a smaller and a bigger wave than us. Sometimes we choose to be small. Sometimes we choose to be big. Either way, we all are still of the same substance. Impermanence is the only constant in life. When life is all over, we will all be part of the same ocean, indefinable and free, one within each other. Remain fluid, but reserve the right to change your mind about anything at any time, because life variables are in constant change. Stay flexible, or the winds of life will uproot you.

Allow yourself to see yourself as you are—a spiritual being present in physical form—and you will not expect yourself to be above or below another human being. Be you, free of roles, hierarchy, and "shoulds." Then you cannot be self-conscious, for what have you to be conscious of if the superficial is swept away? Be yourself: free, equal. Your spirit knows no time, limits, or boundaries. Exercise your essence; float like a cloud. Be true to yourself.

Now, what do you expect from others?

Expectations of others can cause irreversible damage to a relationship, as we become judge and jury to all that is outside ourselves. The news is full of tragedies in which individuals commit horrific crimes precisely because another (or society) did not live up to their expectations. Domestic violence and abuse are also extreme cases of such expectations. It seems easy, in such cases, to identify the victim and perpetrator. Consider, however, that perhaps the greatest victims are the perpetrators themselves. They have made themselves the greatest victims of all. They repeat abuse because they were abused. Abuse is not genetic, it is learned. Abuse begets abuse and is perpetuated by abuse.

Your expectations of others, of course, do not all end up so tragic. Or do they? Is it not a disaster to see a human spirit crushed by another? Is it not a crime to watch a vibrant youth turn into a submissive, conforming adult? Is it not a tragedy to watch one person stifle and smother the individuality of another? Is it not dreadful to be constantly judged? Is it not true that those who judge are often the most miserable people we know? Truly, those who judge cannot enjoy. Herein lies the sadness. Judges, in this sense, become the victims of their own sentences. The real sorrow is that this judge may be you. What does your mirror tell you?

Please answer the following questions to understand how commonplace *expectation/exploitation* is. At first glance, the questions may appear irrelevant to this topic. However, do not look at the arrow but where it is pointing. At the most, the questions may give you insight into your own tendencies; at the very least, they may help you become more aware. Awareness is the first step in any reversal process.

Are you able to willingly suspend your disbelief when watching a movie? Do you find yourself periodically saying to yourself or to others, "This is fake. Like that could happen!" However complicated or simple a task this may be for you, it may well point to your inner propensity to judge. Those who can enjoy the experience of a movie without a continual play-by-play mental judgment may be more likely to enjoy the presence of another without judgment souring the experience as well. Your ability or inability to suspend your disbelief may be an indicator of your ability to enjoy relationships without judgment.

Likewise, do you regularly try different foods? Do you turn down new experiences simply because they are new? Those who typically prejudge an experience or another person or group are unable to fully enjoy. Even turning down a new food without prior experience of it is prejudicial in essence. It is pre-judgment. Prejudice is another form of judgment.

Your inclination to willingly suspend disbelief and your tendencies toward prejudicial behavior and thoughts may be conveyed to your relationships. Can you willingly suspend your disbelief in others? Can their way possibly be the right way? Are others "less" if they are not in accord with your expectations? Is difference palatable? Can you ignore the materialism that surrounds you? As people are sometimes measured by their external worth, this is a valid question. Maybe there is more to life than that. Maybe a person's worth is more than a bunch of zeros behind a dollar sign.

Even those of you who are basically nonjudgmental in nature may be surprised to realize how many times a day you actually make judgments. Try this exercise: Recall one hour of this day during which you were with at least one other person. Now try to remember the events that took place. Who was there? What did you discuss? What did you say? What were you thinking? Please, take this time to write down your answers.

Now analyze your thoughts, actions, and words. Put a check mark by those that were in some way judgmental. How many times did you judge another person? What did you say that transferred your expectation on to someone else? How did you respond when another did not do as you expected? Did you react at all? Were you able to enjoy the presence of others? Or were you preoccupied with your own expectations of what others should or should not do? Are your results alarming? Did you put yourself above the others, below them, or in an equal position?

Remember that we have been raised in a society that is inundated with judgment. We have grown up with it, and it would be a miracle to escape this life view completely. We are eager to label things good or bad, healthy or unhealthy, overweight or thin, superficial or real, industrious or lazy. Even this book may be considered full of judgments. We are a judging society. We judge and are judged.

We cannot escape judging—or judgment—but we can choose to judge in hierarchical terms or in equilateral terms. In hierarchical terms, there is a winner and a loser. In equilateral terms, both sides gain some and lose some as they come to meet in the center, within a mutuality.

Of course, part of being human is our evaluative ability. It separates us from other animals and has been integral in genuine human development. Evaluative judgment, motivated equilaterally, will result in problem solving, creative inspiration, and real connection with other human beings. Evaluation and judgment become destructive, however, when we take our values and beliefs and turn them into daily expectations as we relate with others. Expectations that others live by our rules and behave as we would, make victims. This is expectation exploitation! Eventually, you become your own victim.

Our expectations are born from judgments and the transference of our values and beliefs. Until you know what you believe and value, your expectations may not even be your own—then you become victim to *society's* expectations. However, even when you have successfully come to terms with who you are and what you believe and value, you risk projecting your own values and beliefs onto someone else, especially if that person is someone close to you.

You may expect others to think, value, and believe as you do, and if they don't, there is a problem. Your mission, then, becomes to change or fix that other person to think the way you do. That is simply not completely possible. For those who seem to succeed in "getting" others to act or think somewhat like them, life becomes sadly predictable, lacking life and surprise.

Truly, who of us really wants to be the writer, actor, and audience all at once? Life is wonderful precisely because of the myriad differences and unpredictability. If we write our own life scripts, life becomes a bore.

We become victims of our own expectations. New ideas are curtailed, exciting possibilities are diminished, and our lives are not stretched to new frontiers of understanding. We may end up feeling less dignified or guilty when others *do* as we want. We end up frustrated or even angry when others *do not do* as we want. Either way, we become victims to our own expectations. Either way, we lose.

This is not uncommon. In fact, many people project their expectations on others on a regular basis. Unfortunately, most people do this unconsciously. You can't untie a knot unless you can see it or feel it. You are reading this book in order to enrich your experience of life and to improve your relationships—to become more conscious. We applaud your courage to look at yourself and the way you interact. Your ability to think about your thinking will gift you tremendously. Remember, you are not your thoughts. You are you, merely looking at your thoughts. Please do not confuse your thoughts with your personage, or you will fall victim to your thoughts, cravings, and habits.

Becoming mindful will assist you in letting go of your expectations when interacting with others. It begins with awareness. *We cannot let go of something that we do not even realize we are clinging to.* As you practice just being with another person, you will experience the joy of relationships. It is freeing. Judgments disappear. Enjoyment sets in. Life truly becomes a dance and an appreciation of the diversity that exists. You become a student as you try "first to understand, then to be understood." In this process, you are a receiver, not merely a giver. Mutuality is the essence of a healthy relationship.

How can you truly receive another if you do not willingly suspend your disbelief? Believe in other people's abilities to make their way through their lives the best way they see fit. It is their lives and they have the right to choose and do as they will. They become the architects of their own fortune. (Of course, as parents or primary caregivers, you have a responsibility that goes beyond this as your role dictates a pedagogical responsibility.)

When you put down this book, we invite you to practice *being* in order to become accustomed to suspending your own expectations. When a person enters your life today, slow down and just listen. Listen. Do not attach anything else to your listening. Do not attach your words, examples, or even the nod of your head. Just listen. Be silent. Watch their lips and offer moments of eye contact. Connect. Listen. Let others come into your world. Don't barricade them with your own thoughts and expectations. Don't insult them with your version of their epilogue. Be *with* them.

You may just find them to be sweet nectar to your day or very entertaining. Enjoy others' presence, for there are lessons to be learned. The greatest gift we can give another being is just our presence. Your pet bird, cat, or dog validate that clearly.

Remind yourself that you are a unique person. Celebrate your uniqueness by not wanting another to see life exactly the way you do. Slow down and witness the dance between you and the other person.

However, be aware that others may still project their expectations onto you. Don't get caught up in it. Just watch it. It works! You will be free and full of fun. As you let go of clinging to your expectations, you will be able to watch others' expectations pass by without threat. It may even contagiously inspire others to let go of their expectations, too, and let life into their life. If you become a detached observer of expectations, you will be given a new opportunity to experience gentle humor throughout your day. Like watching a toddler fumble with a football, love for another human being often includes humor. Humor is contradictions and life is full of them. Convert annoyance into private humor. Your humor may mirror your own shortcomings and lead you to genuine compassion. Humor is powerful medicine. Laugh with, not at.

A Circle of Space

Much of what we have discussed leads us naturally into the more specific and habitual positions we take with others, specifically *independence, codependence,* and *interdependence.* Understanding the differences between these three ways of being with others will give you another tool in which to improve your relationships.

Independence

The Fourth of July! Independence Day! This day, we celebrate America's independence from Great Britain. Although this historical event may be a cause for celebration to many in our society, people tend to overapply the value of the very concept of independence.

In fact, our society applauds independence: "Do it by yourself," we are told. "Get out on your own. Be self-reliant." Born out of the need to escape dominance, the independent nature was hailed as an answer and a way into the new world. Although some independent traits *are* honorable, independence can be taken to an extreme. When people believe they do not need others, becoming psychologically independent—an unhealthy, predominant focus on self—sensitivity is lost. Honor is lost. In extreme cases, independent people become totally unaware of those around them, not only physically, but emotionally, spiritually, and mentally, as well. Families suffer when a parent is too independent to participate in the children's lives. Communities suffer when individuals become islands and do not care about the welfare of others. The psychologically independent person loses when she or he misses out on the spiritual dance with others. The extreme of this leads to psychopathic disorders.

Individualism—the belief that the interests of the individual should take precedence over the group—came over on the *Mayflower*. It has taken a foothold here in America. This psychological independence is a preoccupation with one's welfare only, and it results in a loss of compassion and connection.

Look at society today. Neighbors do not relate as they once did. Communities are either too large or too exclusive. Families spend more time away from each other than with each other. In education, sometimes gifted learners are separated so they can learn faster on their own, classes are offered over the computer, and socialization skills are subordinate to the work ethic, all of which applaud the independent learner.

During a 2000 panel discussion regarding *Poverty in America,* Jonathan Kozol, a renowned author and lobbyist, deplored America's indifference to the poverty of children residing in the South Bronx. Receiving $10,000 less per student per year than their counterparts in the elite suburbia next door, children born into poverty have been neglected by our policymakers for too long. Calling our societal neglect the inevitable "theft of the child," Kozol went on to say that Congress repeatedly denies assistance for these impoverished children on the grounds that "independent responsibility" must be society's goal. These children never have a chance. Needing the assistance of a healthy society to interdependently bring them out of the poverty into which they were born, some of these children actually have a greater chance of receiving government aid—at the price of $93,000 per child per year in a prison—than they do of graduating from high school ($8,000 per year per pupil).

The price of independent goal setting is too steep. We cannot afford to abandon our children to the conditions in which they happen to be born. A wolf pack can teach society if we only listen to our brothers and sisters.

Wolves, as sophisticated social animals, care for their young at all costs. Often surrogate parenting and extended families assist when the need arises. How are we as a society doing when considering the plight of our children? Resources need to be invested in our children before they become adults. This gives them a chance and will inevitably reduce the costs of incarceration, addiction, and health care.

Notice that our pattern of independent behavior has been parented by the system of generations past. The hierarchical, male-dominant society begets victims, inequalities, and dominance.

Abuse begets abuse. The invading formula was conquer, exterminate, dominate, exploit, and profit. How much has changed since 1492?

If everyone decided to be independent, chaos would result. Life would become a free-for-all. The quality of life would worsen. Obviously, striving to be totally independent is not the answer.

Where are you in regard to this tendency? Do you need others in your life? Are you aware of those around you? Do you frequently bump into people? Do you notice when someone is feeling bad? Can you ask for help? For directions? Do you *read* the directions? Independent people distract themselves from others. They are primarily inner-world focused and therefore out of balance. In this state, people are more likely to be unaware of any future generation, much less the seventh generation, as self-absorbed blinders restrict the vision necessary to extend oneself beyond oneself.

In fact, independent people are magnets for another unhealthy population—codependent people. In other words, a master needs a slave.

Codependence

Codependency, the other end of the dysfunctional continuum, is a way to distract yourself from yourself. It is predominantly outer-world focused and keeps us out of balance. Codependency has been a hot topic of self-help books, seminars, and therapy for some time. Probably, many people have a basic understanding of what it means to be codependent. Although you may know how it manifests itself, by understanding the system's role in it and recognizing this as the root of the problem, you may free yourself from shame and blame, giving yourself an opportunity to redirect your behaviors and thinking patterns and to consider alternatives to this dysfunctional way of interacting.

Codependency is a word used to describe a component of a dysfunctional relationship. A codependent person is defocused from self, falsely believing that love, security, attention, affection, recognition, approval and acceptance, intimacy, and success depend on *what we do* rather than *who we are.* Think back on what you learned in Part One. Have you come to love your being, who you are becoming, and who you are now? Once you consistently rely on yourself to provide the attention, affection, recognition, and approval you need, even concerning your imperfections, you will more likely break free from this form of relationship. Usually, this means you must do your work with self, striving for balance. What do you need to do for you?

An unhealthy, predominant focus on people, places, and things outside self results in a loss of self-identity. As a codependent person, you give your identity away. You give your power away. No longer do you solely determine how you feel; others now hold the reins that steer your feelings. You allow others to set the mood and tone of your relationships by sacrificing your needs, wants, and aspirations for what you perceive *they* want. You depend upon another to recognize your worthiness when, in truth, you are capable physically and psychologically of providing it for yourself. Thus, codependency results.

Beyond giving his or her own power away, the codependent person takes on accountability for another person. The codependent person may feel responsible for others' behavior and feelings, as the boundaries between self and other are no longer clear. As a servant anticipates a master's needs and complies with the master's desires, so does a codependent person gravitate toward compulsively attending to the other. Within codependency, our inner self diminishes proportionately as we accommodate more and more of the other's expectations. Psychologically, there is no space between the two.

Picture two playing cards that lean up against each other to stand. Like these cards, codependent people psychologically and emotionally cannot stand on their own feet. They come together to brace each other. Along comes stress, which blows onto the fragile relationship and causes it to collapse. He'll blame her and she'll blame him, when, in fact, the relationship was doomed from the very beginning. Their psychological and emotional states created a faulty foundation.

This process leads us to devalue ourselves because we use other people's yardsticks to measure our self-worth. Instead of allowing expression of our interests and feelings, it promotes indirect communication. It makes our own needs, wants, and aspirations secondary. This self-erosion process breeds power-lessness and hopelessness, creating an environment in which many psychological and emotional disorders can flourish. Not taking care of self leads to a compensatory need to take care of others, which fosters a need to control others. This perspective leads to a very serious, rigid, black-and-white viewpoint of the world. But life is not black and white; it's gray.

Codependent people sacrifice self-interest in order to accommodate others. They lose themselves in the process. This self-destructive process leaves them personally vacant. Fear, insecurities, and shame fill the void. This inadequacy and negativity promote anger, resentment, guilt, anxiety, and remorse. It is a self-judging, shame-based existence that lowers self-esteem and self-worth.

This leads to difficulties in identifying personal emotions and a further inability to express emotions in a healthy way. As self-esteem and self-worth decline, the codependent person tries to do things perfectly to prove to self and others that he or she is adequate and worthwhile. Living by a rigid rule system and striving for perfection, the codependent person sets him- or herself up for further disappointment. The cycle continues.

Are you a hostage in this system? Do you know someone who is? More than likely, you or someone close to you is co-dependent. Hierarchical structures and abusive or neglectful homes promote this behavioral response. If this profile fits you, you must not add more shame and blame on to yourself or others. It is time to escape from the downward spiral of shame and blame. It is time to recognize this tendency for what it is: a byproduct of society's teachings. You must add value to yourself, not devalue yourself.

Please take this time to determine if you have any codependent tendencies. Codependency thrives on rules that permeate the system. Some of them may sound familiar: Don't be different. Don't be selfish. Keep deep family secrets. It's only okay for kids to play. If you don't have anything good to say, don't say anything. Don't talk about problems. Don't express your feelings. Don't trust others.

Do you plead guilty to having obeyed any of these? Or do you just *feel* guilty? That's another symptom of codependency.

These negative rules won't allow the expression of one's inner experience, which leads to repression, suppression, denial and delusion. This will make and keep you very sick. These rules are not genetic; they are learned. Given this, you can *relearn* healthy rules and discard the toxic rules. You do not have to be held captive by your childhood. The rules can be changed, and the open expression of your thoughts, feelings, needs, and wants can become paramount. Health and happiness can be found by returning to self-consciousness.

Please understand that what we are talking about here is distinct from genuine caring behaviors. Codependency is an obsessive attachment; caring is a compassionate response to others in need. Codependency clings. Caring does not.

How do you relate with significant others in your life? Is there a healthy space between you? Do you identify and own your feelings? Does the quality of your day depend on what another person is feeling? Does the other person in the relationship set the mood, and do you only react to that mood? Where does your power reside? Are you a perfectionist? Do you regularly shame or blame yourself or others? What do you do for yourself that promotes your emotional, physical, mental, and spiritual growth? There is a need to challenge your codependent beliefs and identify a replacement value system based on interdependence.

Interdependence

We witness interdependent relationships when crisis hits. Floods, tornadoes, earthquakes, hurricanes, and fires seem to bring out our instinctual need to behave in healthy, interdependent ways. We are there for each other. We support one another. We provide the resources necessary for others to get back on their feet. We respect individuals' needs to become self-reliant. We accept help and give help without strings attached.

Why, then, is it such a difficult balance to maintain in our daily lives? Why don't we behave in ways that are instinctually interdependent on any given day? The answer lies in our comfort with the ordinary, our comfort with learned behaviors. Crisis expands our comfort zone; the ordinary stifles it. We have become comfortable with dysfunction.

As you develop interdependent relationships, it is vital to recognize signs of healthy balance between two or more people. In healthy, intimate relationships, space or a degree of separateness is established with one another. Interdependence is not dependent, codependent, or independent. Interdependency allows each person the right to be fully him- or herself without expectations or dominance eclipsing individual growth. Love flourishes in this system, as the space between provides the opportunity for true exchange.

Interdependence signifies a healthy relationship. Our instinctual need for companionship is first highlighted by equality, along with a sense of space between two loving spirits.

The circle is recognized worldwide as a symbol of spiritual power. To be interdependent, two or more people honor the premise of the circle of life. As we each travel on the perimeter of the life circle, we come to see that no point on the circumference is closer to the center of life than another. In crisis situations, we recognize this as we instinctually honor our humanness first. We are equals. There is no hierarchy, only equality. From this point of departure, all other characteristics of interdependence are possible. No one is more. No one is less.

People of equality are often friends. Are you friends with your mate? Are you friends with your children? Do you like them, and do they like you? Are you friends with your parents and siblings? Are you friends with your co-workers? Are you friends with your boss? Why not? Instead of working *for* your boss, work *with* your boss. Some may argue that it is not healthy to be friends with certain people (such as your children or your boss). We disagree. We like our children. Although being parents requires a teaching role for a time, please remember not to confuse that role with who you are. As your children mature, shift your relationship with them from a parent-child relationship to an adult-adult relationship. On one level, you may indeed have a position of authority; however, on another level, at appropriate times, it is vital that we nurture friendships with all who inhabit the earth with us.

Although friendship is ideal, obvious exceptions sometimes make this relationship impossible. Our point here is to encourage you not to rule out the possibilities of friendship simply because of the roles we play. Friendship implies a relationship among equals. You are no more and no less than your children or your boss. We urge you to consider your relationships with all those in your life. Are you friends? And if friendship is impossible, are you equals?

Friendship promotes compatibility. Are you compatible with those in your life? Especially in relation to your partner, it is easy to be interdependent with another when you have common interests. Sports, games, and common projects often bring out this compatibility among loves. Discover what you have in common with those in your life and build off of this bridge. Deliberately plan ways to promote your compatibility. Have fun together.

Compatibility encourages sharing. Sharing is the ultimate act of love and caring. Share your resources and each other. What can you honestly offer another? What are your gifts, your talents, and your understandings? Through exchange and offering, we honor the other.

Sharing includes support. Support one another in your interdependent relationships. Give your presence and validations. Support each other physically and emotionally, as needs arise. The support given and received in your relationship will strengthen you both, together. Honor one another with the support that the other would appreciate when fulfilling dreams and commitments. Let your support for the other be strengthening and dignifying.

Support will nourish your relationship, making the other more, not less. Add value to your relationship, rather than devalue it. Assertive communication, the subject of the next section, will absolutely add substance to your relationship. Communicate your mind and your heart. Respect aloneness as well as togetherness.

Finally, nourishment will promote trust. When you trust and

are trusted, a healthy, functional relationship can grow. Trust is the rich soil that nourishes relationships.

Look to nature to see what works. Red pines, white pines, black walnuts, and yellow birch trees can all inhabit the same forest. Differences are honored and a sense of space separates the circular growth of each tree. Needing approximately an eight-foot separation, each tree grows into its potential. The beauty of the forest exists because of this space and uniqueness. Together, they become a greater being.

Let a sense of solitude define your unique beauty and love, too. Respect the space that allows each individual to author and own her or his unique perspectives, beliefs, values, feelings, attitudes, and choices.

Exercise

Take this time, right now, to author yourself in regard to others. Please write down who you believe you are, what your values and choices are, how you feel and live. Consider, first, just yourself. Be as detailed as you possibly can. Give examples and ground your abstract thinking in something tangible. How are you going to uphold your beliefs and values? What will you do? What will you make time for? When? What options do you have? Which will you explore? When? By creating your circle of separateness, you will add value to your relationships.

———

Now, look at your personal track. Which of your thoughts and attitudes break away from your upbringing? Which are new? Which parallel those earlier values? Do not judge them as right or wrong, just be aware of them. You do not have to discard anything that genuinely makes you more. It is simply vital that you begin to separate others' expectations from your own. Practice being mindful of what is you and what is not you. Practice recognizing when a parental recording is playing through your mind and when your mind is actually doing the recording. What thoughts are really new? What thoughts are really your own? Practice listening to yourself in order to fully be yourself. It begins with awareness.

Now, consider the other person in your relationship. Looking back at what you just wrote, can you see that the other person is not the author or judge of what you have decided? Can you see that the other person is also not the actor of your script? Can you see that in order for you to engage in a healthy, functional relationship, you need to bring *you* to the relationship and not the ideas and values of someone else? You must also honor others for their own life path and decisions. Let go of your expectations and rules.

Break free from the bondage of the abusive system and add value, rather than devalue. Reserve the space between you and your mate, so that your love will have a chance to grow. Let go in order to love in total.

Declare the following disposition:

> I accept you and myself just the way we are. You maintain your destiny through your choices, and I maintain my destiny through my choices. I will not try to change you, and I will not be controlled by you because that constitutes abuse in the sense that abuse is not accepting people, places, and things as they really are. I will encourage you to express your uniqueness, and I will tolerate your differences. I will, however, tell you in an open, honest, direct, calm, and specific manner when you have disappointed me or hurt my feelings. I will state my limits without feeling guilty. I will tell you of my heart and my mind, otherwise you will never know

that of me, and I will only know that part of myself that I share with you. I hope you will share your inner world with me so that I will know you better. I will respond to what I hear you tell me, from your mind and your heart. I will gently care for your honest sharing. Together, may we freely live our lives and commit to one another our love.

Today, this week, this month, and this year, practice mindfulness concerning how you interact with others. Ask yourself the questions introduced so far in this chapter. Take one question a day and allow that to be a guiding point of reference for that day. Do not try to become perfect in a day. That will only happen when you die.

Live each day with a sense of inner freedom. Interdependence is a system in which people can move freely in and out at their will. Self-exploration and personal aspirations are accepted as part of life's path. There is an open, even flow in your new, healthy system. While the codependent person comes from an enmeshed system, and the independent person comes from a distant, autonomous system, your new system is noncontrolling and free. Interdependence is honoring and honorable.

Interdependence is bringing your warrior and your peace side together. The next section will address this new congruency. With an open mind and heart, allow the freedom to be you, free others to be themselves, move your day with joy, and release!

The Middle Road

Walking the shoreline that directs you to a beautiful sunset requires taking the steps to experience fulfillment. It may require strength. You may become unbalanced at times. Painful reminders may accompany your efforts. However, know that each step may also reward you with refreshing delight and a spectacular view for your future. Dedicate yourself to what it takes. Step by step, create and maintain a healthy balance within your relationships with the mindfulness that is required. Walk your sun trail with dignity, pride, honor, and respect.

Perhaps you have now become aware of your expectations of others or the codependent or independent characteristics you learned as a child. Continue to work through these issues as you build meaningful and lasting relationships. Lifelong issues require your attention and commitment. Know this, but also realize that you will grow and improve your relationships with others. Until you are prepared to build a relationship with solid understandings and practices, the most you can do is build castles of sand.

A healthy balance within a relationship is also determined by how one responds to another human being. Passive, aggressive, and assertive tendencies each produce very different results. Passive and aggressive tendencies produce reactions in others; assertion promotes responses. Truly, we teach others how we wish to be treated. Others quickly learn where our boundaries are and what we will and will not tolerate. Truly, as we go, they go. We set the pace. Passive and aggressive tendencies may create codependent and independent relationships. Assertive tendencies are characteristic of interdependent relationships. As each tendency is discussed, try to imagine the role it plays in dysfunctional relationships. It will become clear.

Passivity

Passivity is conflict avoided. Passivity is shutting down, turning inward. Instead of responding to an action or words, a passive person tends to repress or suppress feelings and ideas. Passivity is not speaking up: not saying anything or saying very little. Passivity is accepting or submitting without objection or resistance. Generally, when we think of a passive person, we envision someone who poses no apparent threat, and, indeed, some passive people live out their lives with little outside conflict.

Passivity, however, may be experienced in various degrees and may even alternate with aggressive tendencies. Some may even misinterpret passivity as just being nice. As suppressed feelings build up, however, the person may eventually explode. A passive-aggressive disposition may be born of conflict avoided.

People who always try to avoid conflict actually perpetuate conflict. As values are not followed and honored, the passive person turns this incongruence inward and ends up in a state of internal conflict. Out of habitual people-pleasing tendencies, these people avoid conflict at all costs. Unfortunately, by avoiding conflict, they end up in conflict with themselves. They inflict pain inward at the cost of themselves, abusing themselves.

Whereas extreme passivity (or anger turned inward) may result in suicide, extreme aggression (or anger turned outward) may result in homicide. One extreme is just as unhealthy as the other.

Aggression

Aggression is conflict created. With physical, emotional, or verbal intimidation, an aggressive person is able to get his or her way in a conflict. Aggression is a learned behavior that works because it is forceful power and control. People with aggressive tendencies were taught these behaviors from a significant other or from society. Generally, a person lacking internal power will compensate by struggling to gain external power. Low self-esteem and feelings of insecurity generate this tendency, as they do in the passive person. Temper tantrums—"I want what I want when I want it! And I want it right now!"—may be appropriate during the "terrible twos," but not in adulthood.

People who are aggressive are generally very unhappy inside and subconsciously want others to share in their pain. They turn their pain inside out at the expense of those nearby, or they abuse others. As the adage goes, misery does love company.

Through this discussion, please recognize that one extreme is just as unhealthy as the other. Passivity and aggression are the same thing, just turned inside out, like a reversible jacket.

Please take this time to reflect upon your own tendencies. Do you speak up? Do you effectively communicate your needs and wants? Do you verbalize your feelings? Do you shut down and run away? Alternatively, do you emotionally attack? Verbally attack? Physically attack? Do you bulldoze your way through life? Do you want what you want when you want it—right now? Do you enjoy seeing others squirm? Do you respect and honor others' ideas and needs? Do you see yourself as most important, least important, or equally important? Do you know yourself? Can you be yourself?

As on a seesaw, there is a balancing point between these two extremes, a middle road of peace and health. If you are not balanced, we invite you to make your way to the middle. This will not be a once-in-a-lifetime adjustment. When you find yourself out of balance again, go back to the teachings, push the "reset" button, and come back into balance. Expect that you will need to push your reset button repeatedly, for that is what being human is all about. For thousands of years, many different spiritual practices have acclaimed the middle road as the way to health and happiness. This is not a coincidence. Find the middle and come back to it repeatedly. Equilibrium promotes health and happiness.

Assertion

The fulcrum between passivity and aggression is assertion. The assertive person is someone who seems, intuitively, to come to understand others and be understood. However, assertive skills may be learned. Just as you can nurture an interdependent relationship, you can also learn to be assertive and shed passive or aggressive tendencies. In fact, assertive communication nurtures interdependence. Interdependence and assertive skills both take the middle way. If you learn to become assertive, you will have no further need to retain passive or aggressive tendencies. We retain dysfunctional skills only as long as we do not have a functional replacement system.

Assertive people are easily recognizable. In charge of self, they realize that the only people they can effectively change are themselves. Having truly accepted these limits, they live life as they wear a loose garment, no longer threatened by what others do or do not do. Freed from the need to try to change others, their expectations melt away, and this now-vacated space quickly fills with enjoyment. Assertive people are happy. They are less stressed. They are fun to be around, as they spend their time and energy wisely, balancing their life with health-mindedness. They experience pain and proactively deal with it inside and out—at the cost of no one—as they honor and respect self and others. They also accept pain as an integral part of their life experience. Pain becomes a companion.

The aggressive person fights; the passive person freezes or flees; the assertive person flows. In the *here now*, assertive people are able to embrace the moment. They go with the flow and recognize what they can and cannot influence. They do not push, nor run. They are present with the present, in the present. They yield.

What distinguishes assertive people, especially, are the skills they have acquired. To be assertive means to be *open, honest, direct, calm,* and *specific.* Assertive people communicate very effectively. They express their needs and then are able to detach from the results. They are not clingers. They accept the things they cannot change.

To be *open* is to be ready to receive and give. Those who are preoccupied with expectations and personal agendas are too busy conniving ways to get what they want. Assertive people, on the other hand, welcome new ideas, relish the opportunity to expand their comfort zone, and are free to change themselves in the process. Openness is a soft invitation for others to express themselves in a nonthreatening environment. Openness is like pollen to the bee, sweet nectar to come near. People feel safe in the presence of an open-minded person. To be open is a two-way street. Let others see into you as you see into them. *To be open is to be as expansive as the sky.*

Honesty is the clear transparency over a person's spirit. Those who are truly honest have learned to practice honesty with both the little things and the big things in life. Those who are honest in small ways are capable of being honest in big ways. Honesty promotes trust in others, the foundation of a true relationship. If I cannot trust you, why would I want to invest time and myself with you? Honesty is tested every moment; to be truly honest, one must be honest with self and others. Honesty creates a place where true dialogue begins. *To be honest is to be as deep as the ocean.*

Directness is the ability to say what you mean and mean what you say. Without beating around the bush or forever circling the issue, direct people are clear and concise as they face an issue. They are not time-wasters. Others appreciate direct people, as time is limited. Communication is best when it is clear. As they honor others with the truth, direct people also offer themselves. Direct communication requires commitment and internal direction. *To be direct is to be as clear as a mountain stream.*

Calm is balm to emotional issues and can clear the minds of those involved. Calm generates response, rather than reaction. Calm is an integral aspect of becoming an effectively assertive person. Without calm, a direct and honest person could easily become a bully. Calm diffuses anger and fear; the listener will usually shadow the temperament of a calm speaker. To be calm is to offer a gift of the present, for most negative emotions originate from past regrets or future fears. *To be calm is to be the pause between the breath.*

People who are *specific* can identify and communicate only that which is necessary. Those who are specific do not skirt issues, nor do they leave out important details. Specific information gives the listener grounding, for without it, ideas float away on a breeze. To be specific is to be a good listener first, then respond to what you have heard. The speaker is responsible for what he or she says; however, the listener is responsible for what he or she hears. People who are specific are easy to understand, as they organize their thoughts, express their values, and illuminate solutions. *To be specific is to be the soft sunlight on a shaded forest path.*

Become assertive. Today, practice these five skills, which will promote assertive communication. Like a mantra, repeat, "open, honest, direct, calm, and specific" over and over in your mind as you face relationships with others. If you notice yourself acting passively or aggressively, ask yourself what assertive skill could replace the dysfunction. For example, if you find yourself trying to read your partner's mind, remember to be direct and specific. Ask your partner what she or he means, what she or he is thinking or feeling. If you find yourself bulldozing your ideas onto others, practice openness and the ability to receive others' ideas. Ask for their input.

Pace yourself with all you need to do in redirecting the way you express yourself. What do you have to do today? What is urgent and what is important? Consider what is important, especially if it can become an investment for your future growth and balance. Think before you speak. But do speak! Stand up;

speak up! What do you need to say to others in your life? Say it! Do it calmly, openly, specifically, directly, and honestly. Set limits and boundaries to protect your true feelings and needs. Begin with a plan, know what you need to express, then allow the present to guide your listening. Be open. Be flexible in your listening. Don't expect others to read your mind. Let others know what you need. Only you can advocate for you. *The only one who can help you is you.*

Know that you can say almost anything to anyone in a positive framework. It isn't what you say, but how you say it. Remember this Ojibway teaching, for it will help you in your travels: *Your tongue is to speak with when you know what to say and how to say it. Your teeth are to keep your tongue in your mouth until you figure that out.*

Be open, honest, direct, calm, and specific in your interactions with others and you will achieve balance and respect. Practice these skills with small matters and big matters. Practice them as you would an instrument. Your communication will become soothing to others: a welcomed relief in a frenzied and too-often abusive world. You may also eliminate or diminish negative reactions from others by your mature response. In extending beyond your life circle, you are teaching the future how to communicate. What habits are you sending into the seventh generation? Remember to take the middle road. *Open, honest, direct, calm,* and *specific* are the keys to assertive behavior. Effective communication is the lifeblood of a healthy relationship.

Live and Let Live

Much of what we have discussed so far revolves around ways you can improve your responses to others and strengthen your identity at the same time. Day-to-day stresses and interactions sometimes blur the lines between yourself and another. Unfortunately, those who are unclear of who they are, of the boundaries and space that exist between themselves and another, and their own internal power become more likely to engage in manipulation. Losing sight of who you are and where you begin and end can often lead you into tendencies that are manipulative in nature. Manipulation can become a habit. Ownership and manipulation are major factors in many relationships.

To live and let live is a freeing principle. However, you can only let others live when you have truly learned how to live yourself.

Let live! Let others live their lives. Address your inadequacies, not others'. Take your own inventory, not theirs. Willingly suspend your disbelief. Others do not hold the key to your personal power. You do. What they do or don't do is really none of your business. You are your business. Do not expect, do not manipulate, do not own, do not push. You do not own anyone; this includes their thoughts and their feelings. The only person you have control over is yourself. Allow others to experience their lives the way they decide to. Live your life and let them live theirs.

When you feel inadequate, there is a tendency to manipulate, manufacture, and control to feel sufficient. If you find yourself manipulating, controlling, or giving your power away, your work on self is not complete. The antidote is to continue to work on practices that promote personal satisfaction and self-growth. Go back to Part One and Part Two. Again, the solution is the balance formula.

Live! Those who watch the runners pass by, but complain that their personal energy is low and their weight is high, need to get moving. Change doesn't happen by just thinking about it or watching others work. It happens when you do something about it. Live by doing all that you can to increase your enjoyment of your life. This will require discipline. Just as colors blur at great distances but separate into great distinction as you approach, the true colors of discipline will not be noticeable until time brings you closer to the now-distant goal. Be prepared to exercise patience. Change will not—cannot—happen all at once. Be patient with yourself, but be careful not to use patience as an excuse for inactivity. When you come to know patience, you will then open the door to tolerance.

Discipline yourself to implement your personal formula for balance. What do you need to do today? Do it! Change yourself, inch by inch. Do you need to exercise? Eat healthy? Talk? Read? Pray? Work? Set goals? Give up something? Cry? Play? Do nothing? By doing (or not doing) that which you know you need to do, you actually make future opportunities for enjoyment. Constructive activity will promote constructive results. Success begets success.

Live your life to the fullest. If you knew you only had one hour to live, what would you do? What would be important? Do that! If you knew you only had one week to live, what would you do? Do that! If you knew you only had one month to live, what would you do? Do that! If you knew you only had one year to live, what would you do? Do that! If you knew you only had one life to live, what would you be? Be that.

What do you want your epitaph to read? What's your bottom line?

A healthy balance with others will require you to change. It must begin with you. Shed your expectations, release your dependent tendencies, and learn to implement effective communication skills. Don't expect someone or something to do it for you. The only one that can help you is you! Do what you can—that is all that you can do. Do your best! Enjoy the first steps of creating healthy exchanges with others. This is the groundwork to further fulfillment and love.

Don't worry, don't hurry, do your best, and forget the rest!

Your relationship with others hinges on your relationship with yourself. Others will gravitate toward you if your life is in order, if you enjoy life, and if you have come to balance. They will want what you have. Truly, they may come to you in hopes of catching your enthusiasm for life. This benefits all seven generations, including your own.

Chapter Seven

The Loop of Love

While speaking with Gina's brother a few weeks ago, we entered a discussion on the many faces of God. Gina's brother, an ordained deacon, spoke honestly, honoring the mystery of life. In his open respect for other traditions and beliefs, our dialogue deepened. Here, within an infinite pool of honesty, we connected, not on a religious level, but on a spiritual level. Increasingly, as mystery led to mystery, I realized that the only thing I was absolutely sure of was that I love and I am loved. What a wonderful realization!

You do not need a credential to love. You do not need to be a theologian nor a philosopher. You do not need to be a poet or an artist. You do not need to be a parent or a spouse. You don't need a how-to manual. You simply need to be someone who has loved. You need to have experienced the flow of love, the softness, the joy, the fulfillment of loving another human being. You just need to have loved. It's a natural instinct. It's the greatest and strongest force in the universe. Merge with it, flow with it, become it, sink in it, and soak in it.

Love and Desire

Love has many faces. Look in the mirror.

Many cultures have different words to express different states of love. Love for one's mother, son, friend, or spouse has various shades and is experienced slightly differently. Love for one may accent love for another. Like different pieces of a puzzle, different loves are complementary and make one whole. Still, the core of love is the same, unchangeable, part of the same view. Love's essence is beauty. Love's movement is joy. Love's evidence is tenderness. Love's gift is itself. Love is a free flow of connective energy—a silent vibration of pure delight.

You know you love if you have seen the beauty, felt the joy, experienced the tenderness, given beyond self. If you don't *know* if you're in love, then you're not.

To love another is to offer yourself: your time, your attention, your care. To love another is to offer your strength, honesty, acceptance, and delight. To love is to offer your dignity, pride, respect, and honor.

Ultimately, to love is to be present for another. The greatest gift you can give another is your presence. You do not need to say anything, do anything, be anything. Just be present for those you love in your life. Are you available?

Please take this time now to determine how you will be present for those in your life. What will you do when you put this book down? With whom will you be? Whom will you call? Whom will you join? Engage and be present; offer your love to another.

Go beyond the sentimentality of romance to find the sacred place where eternal love develops. Like a synaptic dance, love between two spirits creates more connections. In the excitement, there is no limit to the love created. Possibilities in love are limitless; hence, your heart can truly overflow. Love is the greatest gift of all; you haven't lived until you've loved.

Know, first, that a space must exist between loved ones. As with neurons firing, if there is no gap, there can be no dance, no creation, no connection. Your relationship with another human being must preserve the space needed for love to flourish. Space allows room to breathe. Respect and honor for the other is integral to developing healthy relationships. Let space join your togetherness. Let togetherness honor the space.

Where are you in this dance with others? Do you love? Have you ever loved? Ultimately, this is what we all look for in another person: someone to love. Our spirit yearns for nourishment. Our spirit yearns to love. Our spirit needs companionship—that's a dominant feature of seven generations; it's all about *we*. We are all one, connected like a spiritual string of pearls.

Listen to the beauty of love as stated in our book *Earth Dance Drum:*

> Love invests itself for itself. Love, although other-conscious, is also self-serving. As we love, we feed our love within. Although two are needed in the exchange, love itself is unchanged, unbroken. Love remembers itself and will urge you toward true loving behaviors. Listen to the voice of love, even when it demands, for love knows what is loving and what is not. Love transcends the experience. True love perpetuates itself, even in the midst of pain, the greed of self, the fear of tomorrow, and the challenge of today.
>
> Love is open, free and spontaneous. Gift yourself . . . a meadow of love. Without time constraints, without preoccupation, without history, love will move you into a wonderful moment. Experience the moment. Love colors the experience with a free flow of energy. Love exists in the now and is evidenced and celebrated with each new moment. . . .
>
> Love is easy. Although situations may be difficult, love itself is easy.

Love for your partner or spouse may come with desire.

Love is freeing and giving. Desire is connecting and receiving. A healthy desire toward your beloved adds passion to your life. Wanting to be near the other, intoxicated with his or her presence, is exciting and fulfilling. It touches bliss. To make love, two spirits create a physical and emotional expression of love or climax release.

Love is the juice. Desire is the fire. But be sure to squeeze. If you don't squeeze, you'll get no juice. Use the juice to spark the fire. Tend your fire well because if you don't, who will?

Desire, distinct from libido or lust, is probably a more accurate word to describe the healthy gravity you experience toward your loved one. Libido infers that you have little, if anything, to say about that which you desire, that you lack control. Lust objectifies the other. The other becomes someone to take or exploit. Desire degrades to lust or libido when respect and love are lacking. Recognize this distinction, become aware of its origin, and you will find the truth.

Desire goes beyond both libido and lust to fill an empty place inside. Desiring your beloved is complementary and exciting. Love, a timeless and spiritual reality, is made physical and experienced in time, through desire. Desire creates, as love imagines.

Become a lover of love. Experience the richness of giving and receiving bliss. It is the balm to our aches, the lift to our wings, the magic to our moments. Love is beyond the songs of the birds or the greatest symphony ever heard. Love is beyond the majesty of the mountains and the eternity of the plains. Love is beyond the gentlest rain and a soothing touch. Love is beyond the sweetest fruit and the smoothest cream. Love is beyond the perfume of the woods and the scent of the rose. Love is our essence. Our spirit is love. We are spirit; we are love. Love is our nature. Love is you; you are love.

Love and desire. What a wonderful life it is!

Love and the Exchange

Too often, people see love and life as something they get or as something they give. Giving is often seen as more noble of the two: better, higher, and other-centered. Getting, often viewed as a self-centered act, is seen as easy and lower. Come to change your thinking. Life and love are not one or the other. They are both. Both may appear one way, but truly be disguised as another. Love and life are to be given and received. Both originate from the heart.

Receiving is distinct from taking. *To truly receive is actually as other-centered as it is self-centered.* To receive with mindfulness, you receive the other person into your life. You are honoring the giver as you receive the gift. In traditional ceremonies, one extends the hands in preparation to receive or waits for the other to offer the item. One never takes it out of the hands of the other. Too often, in today's society, people do not receive. They take without mindfulness of the giver. In this way of thinking, taking *is* self-indulgent and disregards the unique gift of the other.

By truly receiving, being mindful of what the act of giving is about, the receiver lifts the action to the spiritual height that it deserves. Receiving is opening up in order to appreciate that which another gives while honoring the giver. We cannot give without the receiver. The loop of love is reciprocal. Seven generations is also reciprocal, for the first generation is also the seventh of those that came before, and the seventh soon becomes the first.

We can receive (and give) many things that go beyond the material world. In fact, most of what there is to receive truly goes beyond the physical realm. People are eager to give their presence, their words, even their listening, if we provide the opportunity and environment in which to receive.

Children often say, as they learn something new, "Watch this, Mommy!" Eager to share their newfound skill, children give the caregiver a window to their growth. Are we too busy to receive such a gift? What about the playfulness given by one to the other? Playing is a gift of presence and love. Do you receive the playfulness others try to bestow upon you, or do you shrug them off, too busy for such nonsense? Giving feedback is also a wonderful gift another can offer. They offer their perspective. Do you receive their perception, or do you block what they see as unworthy? Too often, we as receivers are too distracted by our own thoughts, our daily preoccupations, and the busy-ness of life to truly attend to what another gives us. To be a receiver, open your mind and your heart. With a grateful heart, one receives.

Giving, on the other hand, is as self-centered as it is other-centered. Giving your attention, thoughts, emotions, objects, and money is an expression of who you are. Give your love; give freely. Open your heart and your attention to those near you. Be present. Give your ability to connect with others. In many tribal societies, a person's wealth is measured by how much they have given away, rather than how much they have amassed—truly a seventh-generation principle.

How often have you received a gift that the giver actually wanted? How often have you given a gift that you actually wanted? In this situation, giving has become nearly totally self-centered. The other has not truly been considered.

Unfortunately, many people today give with strings attached. When you give, do not expect a thank-you card. You do not give for the thanks. If someone accepts your gift in the spirit of appreciation of you and your gift, is that not thanks enough? However, even if that does not occur, and you still expect a thank-you, you need to ask yourself why you gave in the first place. What was your motive for giving?

What has someone gifted you with recently? Are you able to see that most of what is given to you on a daily basis goes beyond the physical realm? Was your heart prepared for the receiving? Did you listen to the heart of the giver? Did you honor the giver? Today, receive the presence of another, the attention of another, the delight of another. Enjoy whom you are with, and you will have received life well.

What have you given recently? Did it come from your heart? Give of your time without conditions attached, without a price tag or expectations. What of your life have you to give another? Can you make room for others in your life? Can you give the gift of space and time? Today, give something of yourself to another in your life. Give your time, your attention, your love. If you cook a meal for your loved ones, cook with the intention of pouring your love into the meal. If you offer a hand, offer it with willingness to extend yourself, in dignity, to the other. If you give a gift, consider the receiver.

Do you give for yourself? Yes. Do you give for others? Yes. Give for both. Receive for both. Life and love are to be given and received like the winds of time, swirling, connecting, moving, and lifting those that they touch. In this way, the receivers of the seventh generation become the givers of truth.

Love and Loss

You *do not* need a credential to appreciate the connection of love and loss. You do not need to be a psychologist or pastor, a doctor or a survivor. You do not even need to have lost someone close to you. Let your heart express what you know of love as you read these words. For, if you have loved, you inevitably know its shadow of loss.

Life is love and life is loss. To love is to risk losing. But not to have loved is the greatest risk of all, the greatest loss of all.

For those of you who have lost someone dear, we honor your silence. Loss resides where no one can enter. In your aloneness, you suffer a love lost. In your silent grief, torment cuts. In your emptiness, nothing is full. Love's shadow has fallen upon you.

To those who have not yet experienced a loss so close, we also honor your silence. For loss awaits in the shadow of your heart. In your aloneness, you suffer imagined loves lost. In your silent step away from grief, torment teases your calm. In your fullness, emptiness is but a moment away. Love's shadow will fall upon you, for the sun must set.

And the sun must rise; life is also love. And to have lived life fully, one must have loved. Therefore, we risk the loss and enter into the arena of love to experience the bliss. Love. As you deepen your relationships with others, you risk loving. As you risk loving, you risk losing. As you risk losing, you risk nothing. As you risk nothing, you come home. Risk and love; come home to your basic self. You will be with yourself for eternity. Better make a friend.

When you love, your immediate feeling is that of gaining the world. Colors look brighter, life is sweeter, holding hands extends further within. Indeed, you gain when you love.

You are more when another enters your life and fills you with their special presence. You are more when you give of yourself to another, for to give is to receive. You are more when you listen to the heart of another human being, for this connects you to your essence, your beginning. You are more when you care for a sick child, for the comfort you offer you also feel. You are more when days are filled with the laughter of those you love, for it spills onto you, and you receive pleasure. You are more when you pray together in love, for your spirits dance the dance of old. You are even more when death takes your loved one away, for their spirit lives on in you and walks with you in your heart.

Love includes the suffering of loss. To love is to gain, but to love is also to lose. We will all experience loss sometime in our life. We will all suffer. We must erode in order to fill and grow again.

Pain will come and pain will go. Love's fragrance transcends the visible world into the mist of the spirit world. Powerful potion it is; it can penetrate the veil of life itself. For your connection to your loved ones who have gone back home to the spirit world is just as strong as it was when they were still on this side.

Suffering, however, is inescapable. It does not simply occur when we experience a final loss of death. Although these losses cannot be matched in pain quotients, loss occurs every day in small ways. Physical pains and emotional pains contain their dose of suffering. Experience and accept small losses in your life, and you will prepare yourself for other losses. Your lungs fill and empty; so also goes your life, in the rhythm of the universe.

Consider the loss you feel after moving, divorcing, leaving friends, changing jobs, watching your children leave home, and feeling your children separate psychologically from you. These are all losses. Grieving that which we love and lose is a natural aspect to living life. Do not struggle against the inevitable. Honor each stage of grieving, for each step brings you closer to peace. That which we fear most reveals what we are. You are made of an infinite pool of love. Love does not end when something or someone ends. It continues. Love is an inextinguishable fire. How sweet it is.

If you love completely, you will understand this: To love is to let go. To live is to let go. Are you willing to let go of your children, to allow them to live their lives separate from you? Do you love them that much? Are you willing to let go of your spouse when you know he or she needs time away? Do you love this way? Are you willing to let go of friends as circumstances change? Can your love survive separation? Are you willing to let go of your parents, your siblings? Can you let go of yourself? Can you let go? If you love all of the people in your life, you must ask yourself this question, for ultimately, we must let go of all those we love. Inevitably, we all must let go. Finally, to love is to let go. The ultimate experience in life and love is death.

To love is to risk losing. To lose is to risk suffering. Fear not; embrace all.

Suffering is our reaction to loss. Negative in connotation, suffering is our way to fight the loss. Buddha said that we all must ultimately let go of our suffering. We must learn to suffer. To suffer is to be human. Suffering is a window to grief.

Expect certain things to happen when you grieve. You may be angry, depressed, in shock. You may bargain in order to try to regain the impermanence of life. Finally, ultimately, you must let go. To let go of what was requires you to honor that which you had. Letting go is not an event. It is a process. Gradually, through anger and sadness, you will work your way toward acceptance and peace. What is, is. Only truth can set you free.

Practice letting go in little ways, and you may prepare yourself to let go in bigger ways. What can you let go of today? How can you practice today?

Suffering is not the final stage in grieving. Acceptance and peace are. New views will eventually fill your day. New loves will fill your heart, and your old loves will nourish their growth. One is not supplanted by another. Indeed, first loves give you strength for risking further love. True love is not limiting, but limitless. Therefore, once you have loved, you are able to love again. You will always be loved because your essence is love. You are love.

Let go. Love again.

The cyclical nature of love and loss is like the seasons in life: first fresh and growing, then mature and beautiful, then gone. So it is with you and your beloved. Experience the exciting growth of new love, for it points to another world. Embrace the colors of love, as they are blissful to behold. Enjoy each moment with your loved ones, as they may be gone the next. Become one in the moment. That's what seven generations is all about: a cyclical, natural order of things that moves from one season to the next.

As you honor each relationship, recognize its sacred mission: to fill you with love. Know and fill up with the love of which you are certain. Take love with you to eternity. Spread love into the seventh generation. Love and be loved. That is the highest gift you can give another. Leave love tracks in the snows of life for those to come to follow.

Love and the Circle

Rub your arms, comb your hair, and notice that you have changed. Skin sheds, hair falls out, pounds are lost. Still, you remain. You are constantly experiencing loss, if you only listen and attend to it. You have lost your youth, or perhaps your waist, your energy, your innocence. Still, you remain. Eventually, you may lose your family, your work, your memory, your body. Still, you remain.

Likewise, when you lose someone dear, you soon realize that person is more than a body, thoughts, and emotions. Her or his spirit remains just as you, too, must remain after your death.

Many people report that they feel empty inside after the death of a loved one. Emptiness, however, does not equate forgetting or nonexistence. The empty state is not permanent. Although you may feel empty for a time, eventually, as the spirit lives on—waiting as though in the shadow of the heart—you (or your beloved) fill the empty space with memories and connection. Like a reproduction of cells, the essence of love for another is endless, beyond time and space. Love continues to grow for our loved ones, even in their absence, for they are always present. If we quiet ourselves down, we can hear those we love, somewhat like distant voices. If we listen also with sharp spiritual ears, we can hear the whispers of our ancestors.

To live life is to be a vessel that empties and fills. Our bodies are filled with our spirits, and then they are emptied once again.

Beyond the sorrow of death, we empty ourselves of life every day. In fact, we must empty ourselves if we ever wish to grow. Our stomachs are designed to empty and fill. Those who never let their stomachs empty deny balance and health. Feel hungry! It's okay. In the same manner, your mind, emotions, and spirit are designed to empty and fill. Experience mental hunger, emotional hunger, and spiritual hunger; this, too, is okay. Expect this cycle of life in all that you do. Expect this cycle in love.

To consider life as only something you gain is to deny the very cycle of life itself. Life is gaining and losing, emptying and filling. The cycle promises one after another, replacing one with the other until the end of time. Come to see that emptying is a necessary step toward growth. You must be willing to let go of your own tendencies in order to improve your relationships with others. You must be willing to let go of others in order to be filled with the presence of those in your future. As the tide goes in and out within the ocean, so does your life empty to fill again with love. This cycle is the melody of love.

What have you to empty? Let go of passive or aggressive tendencies. Empty yourself of codependent rules and habits. Free yourself of all those things that prevent you from developing healthy, balanced, loving relationships. We can only fill after we have emptied. Take charge of yourself. Sculpt yourself physically, mentally, spiritually, and emotionally. Come home to yourself. Love yourself!

Empty to fill. Fill to empty. One without the other is a circle incomplete. Engage the circle of life—the cycle of all things—and honor and love those in your path as you open yourself to further growth.

If we are to grow spiritually in life, we must be willing to empty ourselves of our human weaknesses and character defects as we walk toward love. Let go of all that you think you know. What do you *really* know, anyway? When you are empty of ego, only then can you become enlightened. Love knows no ego. Allow the Creator to fill you with divine love and wisdom. Empty to fill, and you will discover the sacredness in your relationships with others. The sacredness will lead you to joy. Joy will lead you to bliss. And bliss will lead you to the seventh-generation river of life, where all rivers merge into one and form the ocean of one consciousness.

Empty yourself and fill with the future generations. Empty the seventh generation into your life today. Love is this way, a circular vision of love for all. Let the ripples begin.

PART FOUR

BALANCING AND RESPECTING YOUR RELATIONSHIPS

Chapter Eight

Mind and Heart

Here we are: Part Four. We hope that, by now, you have learned to shift between inner-world focus and outer-world focus, recognizing your tendencies of avoidance. Likewise, perhaps you have recognized coping mechanisms you formed during your early years, but no longer serve you well. Or perhaps you came to realize a self-defeating role you take on in order to avoid conflict—whether inside or outside yourself. Can you now slow down? Can you stop? Have you stopped? What have you learned about yourself that you hadn't known before you picked up this book? How does it feel to have redesigned a new lifestyle in order to regain balance in your life?

Now that you have found yourself—so that you can become yourself, be yourself, and enjoy yourself—you are truly able to give yourself to the following seven generations. Through your example and your active participation in developing healthy and balanced relationships, you will be putting down tracks for others to follow.

Remember, health is always a question of balance. In Part Four, you will continue your journey of improving your relationships as you focus on developing and maintaining healthy, balanced relationships with others. As a transformed and enlightened individual, you will have the power to influence the change that is so desperately needed in your world. As a social being, you will discover ways to profoundly celebrate life with others.

Your hard work will pay off today and in the future. Joyful and fulfilling moments await your experience. As you practice offering unconditional love and respect to others, you will experience the quiet peacefulness of knowing your beloved intimately. May you come to touch another human being with a sense of oneness. Ultimately, as you do so, you will take the sacred love found in a relationship with another human being back to the spirit world. No matter who goes first, part of them will stay with you and part of you will stay with them. Relationships with others do not end at the grave.

Ah—the miracle of the mind, the mystery of the heart.

We are thinking, evaluating, appreciating, loving people. With our minds and hearts, we explore our inner and outer worlds. Our minds include our intellect, our thoughts, and our ability to communicate and grow. Our hearts connect us beyond ourselves to the mystery of life.

Mindfulness or circular vision includes that which is around us and within us. It is listening and seeing with the heart. It is about intention. It is marveling at the magnificence created and engineered. Although some people may be envious of minds that go beyond the ordinary, most are innately proud of our fellow humans, for they reflect our own dormant abilities and desires. Our ability to create must be celebrated. The ability to pass these teachings from generation to generation is an enormous advantage if *we,* not *me,* is emphasized.

To see that which is unseen (the work of physicists), or to know the unknowable (the work of mystics), or to hear the silent (the work of chemists), or to touch the untouchable (the work of healers), is truly the calling of each of us. Listen to the yearnings of your mind. We all want to see, hear, know, and touch what lies behind the veil. Yet, ultimately, it is at our moment of death that we will finally be escorted completely beyond our current limits. Ironically, it seems that when our ability to communicate about the universe ends, our ability to communicate with the universe begins. What an exciting moment that will be!

Our minds continue to stretch the limits of our current understandings, however. And those who are the first to glimpse, gather, grasp, or grapple with a new mental frontier are sometimes considered eccentric or special. Come to see that we are all eccentric. We are all special. Those of you who are serious in the quest to improve your relationships with all around and within you have taken on this challenge. To listen to your mind is a courageous step—a risk to expand your comfort zone, to see anew, to evolve your own self.

Our minds are not merely computers with digits and programming. Our minds connect to the eternal—that which is beyond calculations and expectations. Expect the unexpected as you come to listen to your mind. Learn to let go of the ordinary, especially as it binds you to unhealthy patterns of interacting that limit rather than expand your ability to see, hear, know, and touch. Learn to color outside the current lines and limits of your mind. Become again like the young child who, with a box of crayons, playfully explores beyond limits and boundaries. Maximize your potential. Let go of dysfunctional ways of relating, as they prevent you from listening to the depths of your mind and the cosmic mind. Listen. Learn to listen to your body: your heartbeat, then your internal organs, then your skin. You can hear the hidden sounds of nature.

Recently, on a fast and vision quest, Blackwolf's heartbeat became so loud when he rested that it was difficult to fall asleep with the pounding of his heart drum. Silence yourself to hear yourself.

With deliberate mindfulness, you will access the music of your heart, as well. Quieting your mind will allow you to listen to your heart. Like the sap of a tree, your heart feeds the physical with spiritual nourishment. Do you listen to what your heart says? Are you living your life in accordance with your desires, or are you living someone else's life? Do you listen to the subtle frequencies of your heart and the love that needs expression and release? Do you engage others in a way that is *more* rather than *less?* Do you add value to yourself and others, or do you devalue self and others? Your heart is about adding value, about honoring, respecting, dignifying, and offering pride. Love is your heart's language. Beyond words and deeds, love simply lifts the giver and receiver to joyful heights. Your heart is gathering spiritual nourishment to bring back home. Want to increase your wealth? Live, love, and value!

Learn to honor the messages of your heart. It, too, knows what is beyond the veil, for that is its beginning. We are all children of the nothingness that exists beyond all this somethingness to which we cling. We all have a future that ultimately calls us home. Attend to your heart, then, for without it you are not complete. It's funny that nothing clings to something and something clings to nothing. But then, many spiritual principles are paradoxes.

Allow the teachings of this chapter to open your view, rather than close it. Allow the exercises to teach you, rather than comfort you. Allow the understandings to find you, rather than assuming you will find them. Become attuned to your heart and mind. Celebrate your humanness, the miracle, the marvelous being that you are. Let your heart and mind be beacons that guide you to new frontiers. Become an active participant in your connection to the eternal—create your own connections and experience your own epiphanies. Your understandings cannot come from our words and experience, but from *your* experience and words.

Open up to the possibilities. Allow this book to guide you to yourself as you explore your relationships with others and your own internal knowledge. Allow these words to carry you into the seven generations of life's spiraling evolutionary process. Heal your sacred relationships with others as the ripples reach out to the shores of the next generations.

As another tool to come into further balance (spiritually, mentally, physically, and emotionally; in work and in play; with 50 percent inner-world focus and 50 percent outer-world focus; being 90 percent in the present, 5 percent in the past, and 5 percent in the future), align your heart and mind in your relationships with others. With deliberate intention, learn to identify your tendencies in these relationships, create a plan of balance, and communicate the messages of your mind and heart to others.

Alignment of Thoughts and Feelings

Sometimes we are flooded with too much external stimuli, as if we were in the middle of a major city. Sometimes we find ourselves yearning for stimulation if we have been isolated for prolonged periods. This happens quite often in rural and desolate areas. Our nature is social, yet we crave, at a very deep level, to be isolated. Is this a paradox? No, just the ebb and flow of life.

As always, healthy people are balanced between their internal and external worlds. The first question to ask yourself, to determine your state of being, is "What percentage am I externally orientated, and what percentage am I internally orientated?" This, of course, becomes a point of reference from which to make necessary adjustments. The ideal is a fifty-fifty balance.

Your mind and heart must have the space of separateness, yet also join in a balanced dance of togetherness, in order to fully function for your benefit *and* society's. We need both. You need both. Your mind needs the stimulation of others' conversations, ideas, and challenges. Your mind also needs the space of reflection, inward analysis, and internal growth. Likewise, your heart needs the excitement of love given and received, just as it needs the silent presence of only yourself and the Creator. Connecting to the spiritual and physical sides of your being, your heart and mind make the journey to the center of who you are.

Balance your heart and mind. Life is not all thinking, nor is it all feeling. Feelings accent your thoughts, just as thoughts direct your feelings. This is not only an external-internal dance. It is also a mind-heart balance. What percentage are you mind-focused, and what percentage are you heart-focused? *You need to strive for balance between your heart and your mind, with others and without others.*

Shift the spotlight from self to others, ground your thinking to your feelings, and see what may have remained hidden. Center yourself. Commit and create a balance in your relationships with others. The chart on page 151 spatially represents the balance to strive for. Notice how mind-focused activities may support spiritual and physical needs. For planning and discipline are directed from one's mind. Likewise, heart-focused intention may complement spiritual and physical exploration. The chart on page 152 will magnify internal and external awareness, especially as it relates to heart and mind. Exercise circular vision of all aspects of yourself with the grounding that comes with your thoughts and emotions. With awareness, align yourself with center as you specifically consider your relationships with others; be equally focused—internally and externally. Recognize how this linear alignment complements the circular balance you have now grown accustomed to implementing.

In a true sense, once you find and maintain your balance between heart and mind internally and externally you will feed both in a conscientious, healthy way. Allow yourself to fill and empty both your mind and heart, thus guiding the physical and spiritual sides of your being to the center.

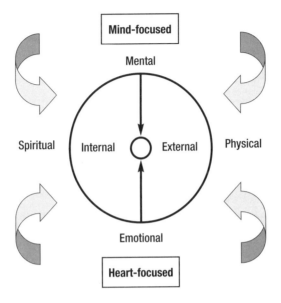

Do not indulge in isolation or social stimulus at the exclusion of the other. Let both your mind and heart empty, and then fill again, in the four areas illustrated on the Mind and Heart Alignment Chart on page 152. Be careful not to starve one or the other, for that leads to imbalance and discord.

Careful attention to yourself will identify your need for others and their need for you. It is our nature to need other people and to form meaningful healthy relationships with them. It is also our nature to form a meaningful relationship with self. One complements the other. To separate your relationship with self from your relationship with others would be like denying the spiritual sap that feeds the physical branches reaching out. Healthy leaves on the tree testify to a balanced system. The leaves of your life evidence your degree of homeostasis.

Exercise

Please take this time to fill in the blank chart below. List today's daily activities and thoughts in the boxes below. You may choose to use the examples that follow as a guide. Note how the physical and spiritual needs for balance are committed with the *intention* of the heart and the mind. Discover how balanced you are internally and externally, between heart and mind. How did you spend your time today?

Mind and Heart Alignment Chart

Strive for Balance	50% Externally focused	50% Internally focused
50% Heart-focused	With others (25%)	With self (25%)
50% Mind-focused	With others (25%)	With self (25%)

Characteristics of being heart-focused with others:
> showing caring behaviors, listening to others' feelings, being with others, playing with others, eating together, expressing intimacy and love, dancing.

Characteristics of being heart-focused with self:
> caring for self (physically, emotionally, and spiritually), listening to and identifying your feelings, reflecting, exploring and being in nature, meditating and praying, taking time alone.

Characteristics of being mind-focused with others:
> working together, discussing and solving problems with others, listening to others' ideas, managing daily life.

Characteristics of being mind-focused with self:
> writing, reading, learning new ideas, expanding comfort zone, identifying and strategizing a personal formula for balance, disciplining the body to exercise, working.

Note: Some activities may fit in more than one cell. Walking with your spouse is heart-focused with both others and self, as you are sharing your company and working on your own physical health. If you solve problems on your walk, it also becomes mind-focused with others.

As you become increasingly comfortable with identifying your tendencies and then working to balance your day, the need for such a chart or tactile reminder will not be necessary. You will automatically come to balance, as do all things in nature. You will begin to balance your life because you will crave the internal harmony that this deliberate attention gives you. Recently, Gina renewed her commitment to physical health by running each morning. After three weeks, she no longer needed the alarm clock (and mental reasoning) to get out of bed in the morning. Now she gets out of bed in the morning because her body naturally craves the health that the exercise gives. However, expect that establishing new routines may be difficult at first. You indeed may need someone to guide and encourage you. We do. That does not show a sign of weakness. Instead, it shows a realistic view of where you are with yourself now. Do what it takes to move yourself in the direction of balance. If you need help, then get help.

Your internal measurement of peace, serenity, and tranquility will become a compass leading you continuously back home to your heart and relished balance. Your serene, placid state will tell you all is well. Your disharmony will let you know what you need to find your equilibrium again. You inherently have all the internal resources you need to actualize this state of being. In other words, when your canoe tips, you need to regain balance, or you're going to get wet.

Listen to Both

Popular music nearly completely focuses on relationships with others, especially in an idealistic sense. Many people grow up romanticizing love. What is love? Why does it hurt? When will it come again? Where does one find the perfect love? Listening to popular music constantly reminds us of our need to connect with others.

Yes, music *is* the language of our spirits. To enjoy the rhythms and the melodies and harmonies can be soothing or invigorating. Music is, of course, wonderful and fulfilling, energizing and beautiful. Such reminders of our need for others are good and often touch a sentimental place in our hearts. But why does our society choose to dominate the airwaves with lyrics that focus on loves lost and gained? As culture reflects the health and balance of the people, what is our culture reflecting? Our insecurities and our imbalance? How many codependent people are there? What needs are these lyrics trying to fill? The lyrics point to a cultural trend. We are a needy society, and the words reflect that reality. Lyrics that state, "Life is not worth living without you," are tragic. Are we not here for our own personal reason? To make another person your reason for living suggests that you do not know of the truth of your beginning and end. Will not your first breath and your last breath be our own? Are you an extension or are you freestanding?

Repetitive messages engrain priorities. Listening to and thinking about one's need for others has the potential to make others a priority over self. Have we nurtured a codependent element to society? Consider the effect of popular music switching its focus completely to self. Perhaps a predominantly independent culture would result. However, we need balance.

Those who balance their listening with alternatives such as classical or instrumental jazz focus on self-connection as well as other-connection. Here, in this example of contemporary music, there is a listening to both aspects of the heart.

What music do you listen to? Are you able to appreciate instrumental music as much as you appreciate lyrical? Likewise, do you ever allow yourself to listen to popular music for its message of the heart? Allow this reflection to point to how you listen. What do you think about? Do you allow the same concerns to monopolize your heart? It is essential that you spend as much time listening to your heart about self as you think about others and vice versa.

Allow friendships and family relationships to teach you about yourself. Listen to the truths reflected back from the people in your life. Oftentimes, what we loathe in another is what we do not like about ourselves. Maneuver between your hopes, dreams, needs, and wants concerning all who live in your heart. Include yourself. Relationships, a mutuality of regard, begin with honesty and end with honesty and love. Sprinkle in respect and integrity, and see how sweet it is!

Listen to your heart. Your heart will honor you, just as it honors those you love. Relationships must carry that special ingredient, love, like yeast in bread. Without love, relationships go flat, never to experience the heights of what is intended. Relationships crest according to the degree of energy invested. You get out of them what you put in. Invest in happiness; it pays dividends.

Just as you listen to your heart, listen also to your mind. Listen to your thoughts, as they guide you in your journey. Your thoughts will reflect your values and priorities. It is essential to allow your thoughts to teach you, as well. Slow down. You will learn about yourself, your tendencies, and how you deal with others if you just listen. There is that voice that urges you to listen. Do not ignore the internal voice; it is wise. It knows what it knows simply because it knows.

Thoughts aren't just thoughts, but signposts of what is going on within you and outside you. Thoughts will warn and beget emotional responses. So be in charge of your thoughts. Who else will be if you are not?

Listen to your thoughts to discover your weaknesses. Learn and grow. Develop understanding and tolerance. Expand your comfort zone with challenges.

What you choose to put into your mind has the potential to help or hurt. Just as what you put in your mouth determines your physical condition, what you put in your mind determines your mental condition. So please remember: What goes in must come out in some manner, whether in the form of bad dreams, emulation, or simply discomfort.

Listen and be mindful of what you allow to access your mind.

As popular music points to codependency, the media now points to abuse. Just as the media reflects the abusive and sexually exploitive nature of our society, it also, in some degree, promotes it. You must determine the fine line between art and exploitive aggression. Listen. You know. It is your responsibility what you put into your mind and no one else's.

No one can change you but you. You are the determining factor. Your spouse, friend, mother, sister, brother, father, daughter, son, psychiatrist, or spiritual guide cannot change you. They certainly may help you, but they cannot change you! Some may claim to read minds and tell your fortune, but they cannot listen to your heart. You can listen to all those you love until they run out of words and still they will not have the power to change you. This book cannot change you. Only *you* can change *you*. Listen to yourself. Listen to your heart and your mind. Listen. Desire is the fuel on the torch of change. *I can't* means *I won't,* and *I can* means *I will!*

Communicate Both

You can measure the quality of a relationship by its level of communication. The quality and quantity of communication determines the direction of a relationship. Those couples and families who have mastered the art of communicating effectively prevent many problems from escalating or even from occurring in the first place. It is vital that you develop the skills of assertive communication with those you love. The results will be trust, empathy, and a deep understanding of each other. Learn to communicate both the concerns of your mind and the concerns of your heart. Learn to listen to yourself and the other. Give and receive openly, honestly, directly, calmly, and specifically. Communication is not a one-way street. It takes two.

A healthy person needs to be able to communicate openly, honestly, directly, calmly, and specifically about issues of substance, concerns, and expectations. For some, it is not threatening to express what is on their minds. Sharing thoughts and ideas, especially if there is no emotional price tag attached and if the recipient is also open, often seems easy. However, it is not automatic.

Many people censor what they say, leaving out details that may instigate an emotional response from the listener. In fact, many people get into relationship problems because they neglect to tell the significant other something of great importance. Often the reason for the omission is "I didn't want to hurt your feelings." Clearly codependent in nature (taking on responsibility for the emotional welfare of the other), this lack of direct communication escalates other relationship problems.

As you know, *it is not what you say, but how you say it.* The assertive formula eases most difficult discussions: Be open, honest, direct, calm, and specific. Reminding yourself of these principles will guide your discussion into understanding. And, at the risk of sounding uncompassionate, even if what you say would end up hurting the other's feelings, so what? *Intention* is the key. Are you intending to hurt or help? It's that simple. Their feelings are *their* feelings, and people can deal with their own emotions. Remember that emotions dissipate with time. I wonder if you can ever do better than telling the truth. As a receiver of negative information, you also need to recognize that you own your feelings and that your emotions will evaporate over time. Don't just view life with your mind; experience life with your emotions, also.

This advice, to communicate freely, also applies to an open expression of feelings, the vital force of our humanness. Here is where many people have difficulty. The first step in expressing your feelings is to identify your feelings. You must know what you feel before you are truly able to express it. Practice identifying your feelings throughout the day, especially if you usually end up angry. Anger is generally a secondary feeling, disguising a more basic feeling. Ask yourself, "Why am I angry?" You may find out that you were hurt, ashamed, afraid, or frustrated. Then embrace that emotion. Feel it, experience it, and it will dissipate itself. The winds come and the winds go. It's just their nature. So go your emotions.

Once you can easily identify your emotions, realize that they are your emotions. No one but you makes you feel anything. Your feelings may have been stimulated by what someone said or did or didn't say or do, but come to see that you own your feelings and that others are not responsible for your feelings. They *are* responsible for what *they* say and do—perhaps something "hurtful"—and it is their responsibility to consider the effects of their actions on others. However, they do not *make* you feel anything. If you were hurt, you need to ask yourself why. What was threatened? Why were you threatened? What could you do to change that perception? Remember, if you place too much power in the hands of the other, you have given your power away. You have allowed another to determine the kind of day you will have. Push your reset button and start your day all over again.

Next, if that other person is more than a casual acquaintance, it may be a good idea to communicate how you feel to that other person so she or he can learn about you and perhaps gain insight into their own behavior. Remember to own your feelings. Use I-statements such as, "I feel hurt that you did not tell me the truth," and you will be less threatening and may open a channel for genuine dialogue. Communicate your feelings.

How can anyone possibly know you if you do not communicate your heart? Please remember that feelings include the "negative" and the "positive." Communicate love. Do you hug? Do you tell those in your life that you love them? Do you regularly remind others just what it is about them that you enjoy? Do you hear the messages of love sent your way? Again, with balance, attend to the communication of your heart but not at the expense of denying other aspects of your being. Ultimately, on our deathbeds, we may all be concerned with the messages of our hearts and whether we adequately expressed our love to those dear to us.

We also need to define and live in accordance with self-determined limits, boundaries, and a sense of direction. You have the right to set limits and boundaries. They reflect your commitment to both your mind and heart.

You are not an open door that must allow whomever and whatever into your life. If someone is living a life that is not in harmony with your own value system, you have the right to insist on separation. Communicate, in an open and direct manner, what you will and will not tolerate. *Remember, you teach others how to treat you.* If you set limits, you have improved the odds that your limits will not be violated. Clearly and specifically communicate your needs. Communicate calmly, and emotional flare-ups may not ignite. It is your life, and you may choose how you will live it, with whom, and with what direction. Do not allow others to determine your day. Determine your own day. Do not allow others to determine your life. Live your own life. Say what you mean; mean what you say. Get a grip, hang on, and hang in there. That's the secret of life. Too simple? Maybe. Too hard? Maybe. Do it anyway. You'll change your life forever.

Just as senders of messages may need guidance, so may receivers. It is vital that you *respond* to others in an open, honest, direct, calm and specific manner. Respond to others' hearts and minds with your own open mind and heart. Do not attach your own values and filtered explanations of what you think they mean. Can you read minds? Do you respond to what others say or rather to what your mind has determined they really meant.

Be direct: Ask if you don't know. Be honest: Don't guess. When you hear another person report, "That isn't what I meant," one or both of you are not communicating (sending *and* receiving) in an open, honest, direct, calm, and specific manner.

What have you communicated with others today? Look at the chart that you filled in earlier. Did you take the opportunity to express your mind and heart? Have you set limits with others in your life? Did you listen to what others were trying to express? Did you hear their hearts and their minds? Practice communicating both your heart and your mind in an open, honest, direct, calm, and specific way, and your relationships with others will improve. How could they not improve? Clear communication is sharing of self and leads to intimacy.

Chapter Nine

Respect All, Fear None

 hen you are with others, where is your attention? Do you attend to only what is going on inside of you? Are you always other-centered, wondering what others are thinking about or feeling? Or are you somewhere in between? The space between is a very healthy place to be. Your growth concerning your relationship with self and others will become evident as you consider your attitude toward others, because attitude begets behavior.

Do you fear others? Do you respect others? These two basic questions can be easily traced back to self. All of our relationships begin with who we are.

If you do not fear yourself, you will fear none. If you can respect yourself, you can respect all.

Some would argue that fear of others has nothing to do with fear of self. Others do intimidate and control. Although this may be true, as we learned in the last chapter, how you respond to their intimidation and control is completely up to you. Fear of others has everything to do with your fear of yourself. Your ability to trust yourself denies others absolute power over you. In charge of your own thoughts and feelings, you are able to extend your hand without fear, for you know who you are and what is important to you. You are protected by your self-worth. Those who give their power away do not exercise internal power. Your attention outside self diminishes your trust of self. Find that secure spot within yourself. If it is not there, then build a comfortable nest within yourself. We are the creators and crafters of our home within our hearts. Is your heart-home comfortable? Or does it still need some design and work?

Likewise, if you are predominately attending within, your ability to extend honor to another lessens, as you are unable to hear and see the contribution of another. *Respect for self includes the instinctual need to connect with others.* Those who do not respect this particular aspect of their being are unable to give others the respect they inherently deserve. When disrespect pervades other areas of your being, you become less and less able to respect others. Your low self-esteem is projected onto those you meet. Unable to respect all aspects of your being, you are unable to respect all aspects of other beings. Intolerance for self results in intolerance for others. Disregard of self promotes disregard of others. Absence begets absence, and emptiness prevails.

If God appeared as a personal God before you right now and told you that you are equal to all who live on this earth, would you believe this? Would you change in the way you approach others?

Respect who you are and trust (do not fear) your abilities to do what is best. Once you believe this, you will be able to extend this respect to others and be free of the fear that too often limits human potential. Doing your best is a degree of competence. No one is perfect. Do not raise the bar beyond your capacity and limitations.

Although confusion and the inability to trust can be traced back to the family system, you can now trust yourself and provide personal stability. Let go of the broken promises, mixed messages, and contradictory information that perhaps led to mixed feelings and the inability to make decisions. Do not allow insecurity to continue to follow you through adulthood. As you continue to work on the self-defeating tendencies that you have identified so far—as you add value to self—remember that the past is past and now is now. Now is your opportunity to create quality relationships with others. Maturity is letting go of self-defeating tendencies. Sometimes it requires you to let go of the past. Keep of your past what is helpful; discard what is hurtful.

This chapter will identify the defense mechanisms that may be interfering with or promoting a continuance of fear and disrespect that you may have for others. Through understanding these techniques—which you learned as a child in order to survive—and finding ways to replace them, your interactions with others will improve. As you continue to honor the diversity of life, and as your respect for others grows, you will be well prepared to leave a legacy for others.

The Dance of Truth

Beyond us lies a vast ocean of people. How we present ourselves will pretty much determine their reactions and responses. To be sure, smiles usually beget smiles, sternness begets sternness, disrespect begets disrespect, and respect begets respect. You might well ask yourself what kind of responses you desire and present yourself in accord with the desired results. Our external circumstance is pretty much determined by our internal circumstance.

Yet, beyond the social mirrors we create, there are many things we cannot change. There are many people with ingrained dysfunctional behavior patterns and habits who are unwilling or unable to do anything about them. The best we can do is to recognize their moves and learn how to appropriately respond. Note that this area of relationships, however, will come in the next section. This section asks you to look at yourself.

Life is full of psychological movements. Some are healthy and fun, playfully honoring others as we dance through life. An emotional and psychological dance with another denotes the ability to connect, respond, and have fun. However, most psychological maneuvers are noticeably dysfunctional and are strategic ways to prevent true intimacy; they are made of fear and disrespect. As we discuss specific tendencies, you may recognize the patterns of someone close to you. Although this information may be helpful, refrain from judging. Instead, keep the focus primarily on you.

Discover which patterns you habitually follow. You may need to change your tune or find a new dance partner. Only you can change you.

Observe your interactions with people, and you will learn about yourself. Observation of your response and another's is a wonderful teaching tool. You may soon discover many techniques people (including yourself) use to avoid the truth. Ironically, what many don't realize is that the truth, if embraced, sets one free. People skip around the truth constantly and believe they deflect the attention that their problems attract. Their intricate steps of memorized movements keep others at an arm's distance. These people are afraid to let someone into the embrace that encloses who they are. Fear of intimacy, rejection, or abandonment issues may also preclude real connections to another human being.

Those who come to another with feelings of inadequacy and low self-worth may also attempt to hide this. They may try to protect their self-image from shame, guilt, anxiety, and fear with defense mechanisms. As a child, you may have had to develop ways to maintain a tolerable version of reality. You practiced these types of manipulation, and eventually you became what you practiced. This psychological camouflage makes the mind believe that things are different than they really are. At the same time, these mechanisms serve as protective coating to conceal truth and avoid responsibility. It's like a magician using mirrors to shape a different version of reality. These tricks become more palatable and comfortable to the user and consequently bolster self-esteem. Nonetheless, these techniques are delusionary. And delusion begets denial.

As one begins to believe these self-delusions, he or she gets further and further away from reality and soon may become hopelessly trapped in self-deceptions. Although movements appear clever and fluid to this person, others may see a disjointed pathetic effort at denial and delusion. Delusion is like putting ink in the water until the self becomes invisible or murky. In the effort to deceive others, we outwit ourselves.

These defenses serve two primary purposes: denial of reality and delusion of the truth. In most cases, these manipulations lead the victim into depression because he or she is living a lie. You can lie to your mind, but not to your heart, so at some deep level you become disturbed.

The following mechanisms may sound familiar to you at some level. Whether they ring a bell or remind you of someone in your life, please continue to look at self in order to change the only person you can—you. These defense mechanisms more than likely are not all that foreign to most of us. We truly are in this together.

Withdrawal is a defense that takes us into ourselves and isolates us from the true validation of our outside world. This shutting out of external reality leads us into an inner fantasy world, which all too often promotes severe mental illness syndromes. Here, we move alone and become progressively distant from self, others, and reality. Some people may simply "check out" or remain aloof. Some people invest no spark or effort and take no responsibility for or ownership of the relationship. They contribute nothing, yet expect everything. These people suck us dry and leave us shells of ourselves. Perhaps you know people like this. Do what you have to do to maintain your health, or they will deflate you.

Rationalization involves the manufacturing of reasons why we do things instead of examining the real reasons. We try to sidestep the truth with self-convincing false rationale, which distorts reality and traps us in our illusion. A litany of excuses results, and life then becomes a series of mental push-ups that takes us further and further away from truth. Afraid to speak the truth, we lie with simple or outlandish justifications.

Projection is a technique in which we turn the spotlight away from our self and onto another person, place, or thing. We make them responsible for our actions and do not hold ourselves accountable. All too often, we take what we don't like about ourselves and attribute it to others. Through shadow puppetry, we avoid the truth of self, blaming others and attributing our most negative attributes to others.

Compliance bends us to accommodate others, even though it may compromise our values, beliefs, and integrity. Compliant partners do not want to make waves and will invest a great amount of effort into avoiding conflict. The problem here is, by avoiding external conflict with others, we end up in internal conflict with ourselves because we have compromised our personal principles. We have disrespected self. When our behaviors are in conflict with our values, we become out of balance, and pathology emerges. Frustration then ensues, and prolonged frustration converts itself into anger. Prolonged anger converts itself into resentments, which fuel and perpetuate anger. You may have witnessed this in other people. They are easily angered. Their fire may smolder at times or explode into rage. It, too, is sparked from denial and delusion. It's flammable stuff.

Minimizing erases the outer borders of a picture until the core image is barely visible. We make something truly significant into something insignificant. We mentally devalue a person, place, thing, or event to a trivial point, reshaping its truth to fit our thinking. "It's no big deal," we tell ourselves, when in fact, it is! It is what it is.

Many people often engage in *agreeing,* another defense mechanism. We betray ourselves when we agree with others, knowing we have compromised the truth. This maneuver may well eliminate external stress, only to develop internal tension and falsehood, which forces us to live in an internal hostile environment. This leads to internal incongruence. As a great breeding ground for guilt, remorse, and shame, this mechanism not only chews us up, but will depress us as well.

Verbalizing is a technique in which a continuous flow of trivial conversation is activated in an effort to avoid issues of substance and emotional rapport. This fancy footwork avoids the truth at all costs. Our vocabulary may improve at the expense of emotional intimacy—truly a price beyond comprehension. When we defensively verbalize, we are afraid of being open, honest, direct, calm, and specific. We are avoiding, thereby not being assertive.

Finally, there is *denial,* the outright refusal to accept something about ourselves that is unpleasant. This is like stepping onto quicksand. People who follow this technique are sucked into the abyss of denial. Everyone else knows they're living a lie. The sad part is that they have contrived and now believe their own myth.

If you recognize yourself in any of the defense mechanisms that were described, it is up to you to change your steps. The anecdote is obviously to address the truth and to see things as they really are. Constantly ask yourself if you are being honest. Continue to walk through your fears. Lay your cards on the table and turn them face up. In this way, you are respecting yourself and others to deal with the truth.

A helpful hint: With brutal honesty, ask yourself, "What is my *motive* for avoiding the truth?" The motive is the mirror of truth. This avoidance is the catalyst for your denial and delusion, which, of course, will definitely lead to depression. It's depressing to live a lie. And it's freeing to live the truth!

Do not fear your ability to deal with the truth, and you will not fear others' responses. Trust yourself. Respect all; fear none. Dance the dance of truth—dancing is fun.

When dealing with others' defense mechanisms, we need to confront the behavior, not the person. The next section will give you further insight into dealing with others.

Colleagues, Critics, and Competition

Much of our life at work may require us to interact with people who flit around truth on a daily basis. Although you cannot change others, you can influence your work environment by the precedents you set. Effective working relationships flourish with unified respect, assertive communication, a sense of trust, and cooperation.

Interdependent relationships at work must begin with the same prerequisites of all interdependent relationships: equality. Working with a team of people must begin with an open discussion of one and only one expectation: respect. We don't even have to like one another to have a healthy relationship; however, we need to respect one another.

What you say and how you say it may very well facilitate genuine proactive dialogue among co-workers. You must continually exercise assertive communication, being consciously aware of your habitual tendency to be perhaps aggressive, passive, or passive-aggressive. Remember, your habits go with you. Practice speaking to your colleagues in an open, honest, direct, calm, and specific manner. It works! By not denying reality or deluding the truth, you can set a precedent. Others may follow your example. Your forthrightness—respecting others and fearing none—may result in your colleagues, in turn, respecting you. The more you practice these principles in all your affairs, the healthier your relationships will become.

Criticizing, complaining, gossiping, and belittling are commonplace in work environments. Unfortunately, much of this is done in secrecy. Even if you are not the target today, you may become the lightning rod tomorrow. You may well think, "How can I trust? Will I be next?"

Trust within a profession and trust among different professionals can only occur if respect is unanimously given to each other. This does not mean you need to agree with or condone all that others do. You can respect others even if you disagree with their ethics, behaviors, and decisions. Within an intellectual discussion, we don't always have to agree. With your assertive skills, confront problem co-workers; don't talk behind their backs. Fear none. What is the worst thing that can happen? Your knees shake and your voice trembles? Then shake and tremble. They'll get angry? Let others deal with their own emotions. Whatever happens, at least you have been true to yourself. Remember, by avoiding conflict with others, we end up in conflict with self. What is the best thing that can happen? Perhaps an open dialogue and genuine understanding. Express your needs, wants, and comments. If appropriate, express your dissatisfaction. Directly relay one person to another if issues arise. Do not speak for someone else. Respect all by assertively communicating only what is yours to communicate.

Perhaps there is someone in your work life whom you have a difficult time getting along with. Communicate assertively and encourage that respect be given to all. Do not deny the truth—set yourself free. Be it, say it, walk it, live it.

Just as trust and respect enhance relationships, so does cooperation. Cooperation is energy directed in unison toward a common goal. Write a common mission statement, decide on a common goal, and combine your efforts. Become like a centipede; in a tug-of-war, the side that uses the centipede principle, with all legs working in unison, wins. Become of one mind. Together, create a win-win vision, rather than a win-lose dilemma or a competition.

Competition sours relationships. And soured relationships interfere with and diminish productivity. In the workplace, co-operation is constructive, while competition is destructive. Let's look at business. Businesses function to make money. Unfortunately, some are profit-driven organizations that make money at the expense of professional ethics. For example, some health maintenance organizations are currently being criticized for this very reason. The voice of the people is being heard via the Patients' Bill of Rights. We can learn a lesson from this example. Don't allow economics to supersede professionalism. Do the right thing and money will follow. Ultimately, soured relationships sour society.

Money is like water: There is dirty, polluted money that is gained at the exploitation of people and nature. And there is pure, clean money, which is gathered and harvested without polluting nature or exploiting people. We invite you to review your investment portfolio to see if the companies you have invested in are generating clean or dirty profits. You may want to make some changes. Your relationship with money may bring a new dimension to your conscience.

Different Paths

How many people do you know fairly well? Twenty? One hundred? Five hundred? How many of them are from a different cultural upbringing? How many speak another language fluently?

How many are of a different color? How many of your acquaintances have a different religious background than you? How many believe in a different *world* religion? How many of them work in a very different field than you? How many of your acquaintances are at a significantly different economic level than you are? How many acquaintances, other than relatives, live outside a fifty-mile radius of your home? Now please go back to your first answer. Out of all of your acquaintances, how many people would you consider significantly different than you? Ten, five, two, none? Of these, how many do you know very well? How well do you know their values, beliefs, fears, hopes, and dreams?

Some of you may come up with numbers that evidence a very diverse upbringing. Perhaps you lived in a multicultural epicenter during your formative years. Perhaps you know many people from different cultural, religious, and economic backgrounds. If you are of this minority, you may indeed have a great ability to relate and appreciate differences in others.

Most of you, however, probably have a low number that represents your limited extension into our diverse world. Perhaps, due to your predominant hometown culture, you never had the opportunity to learn about different people and how they see life outside of what you have seen on television, read, or heard on the radio.

Although this seems obvious, many people avoid the fact that *where* we are born determines much of our external paths. Luck and circumstance do play a role in what religion you will die for, what socioeconomic status you hold, what prejudices you will carry on, what cultures you will be acquainted with, what traditions you will continue, and even—to some extent—what future is possible for you. You are, to a significant degree, a result of your birthplace and circumstance.

Many people born into poverty will never escape poverty. Many born into a dominant cultural legacy will never go beyond that which is passed down. Many born into abusive homes struggle to end the cycle; some will, but many will not. Many born into limiting perspectives never dare stretch their minds to encompass other potential ideas, philosophies, and even religions. Limits innately accompany any cultural background. We all grow up limited in one way or another.

Exercise

Please do this next exercise with as much honesty as you are able to gather. Please pause after each question and write down your initial response. Consider your life, had circumstances been different. What would you be like if you had been born into a wealthy home, a poor home? What would you be like if you had been born into an Islamic home, a Catholic home, a Jewish home, or a home of indigenous beliefs? What would you be like if you had been born into a dysfunctional and abusive home, a functional and supportive home? How would your life be different? How would *you* be different? What version of reality would you subscribe to?

These are important questions to ask, as there are indeed many paths in life. On what path did you begin your life? Your external path has the potential to control your internal path. The relationships you avoid or are attracted to may very well grow out of your birth circumstances, your comfort zone. If you doubt this, please answer the following question: Which of your beliefs and values are more than simply consequences or natural outgrowths of the path on which you began your life? For example, is your religion your parents' religion? Is your hometown your parents' hometown? Is your food preference your parents' food preference? Did you follow in the family's business? Does your tolerance reflect your parents' tolerance?

If you were unable to name even one attribute or characteristic that seems uniquely yours, you are certainly not alone. Most of us are nearly the sum total of our experiences and circumstances. (Of course, our total being is greater than the sum of our parts, because we have our spirit, which encompasses us. We are a spirit with a body, not a body with a spirit. However, the parts we are now discussing do matter in your life direction.)

What we do with our individual experiences and circumstances needs to be our focus. If you never reflect upon that which is externally promoted in your life and distinguish it from that which is internally promoted in your life, you will always be a victim of your own circumstances. Those who are able to look at their circumstances, and see them as exactly that, are free to free themselves of the conditions and limits that naturally accompany their original life path. This is risky business.

Consciously evaluating what you have automatically accepted your entire life is like beginning a controlled fire. What if it gets out of hand? What if we destroy everything that is who we are? Then we need to review who we really are.

You are a spiritual being temporarily experiencing the physical dimension with a body, mind, heart, and spirit, who is here to "live, learn, love, and leave a legacy."

In no way are we suggesting that you get rid of your beliefs and values, your religious training, money, or work. That would be foolish. We need to accept our individuality, for it is our differences that make us unique from all others and provide us with opportunities for our continuous growth, both internally and socially. Roots are needed.

What we *are* suggesting is that you open your vista to the rest of the world with equal respect and honor. Look at yourself from a global perspective, rather than simply a hometown perspective.

In doing so, you will be able to see others with a softer, more circular vision, as well. Learn to listen with your eyes and see with your ears. Learn to use your senses in different and developed ways, like blind and deaf people often do.

Your spirit eye will tell your heart things that are not available to you through any other means. It's the strong spiritual cord that strands the seven generations together. Handed from one to the next, the torch is perpetually passed.

Just as your life path can lead you to truth and love, so can other paths lead others to truth and love. Different paths are just that: different, but valid all the same. Once you come to see that diversity is the color and richness of life, you will be able to let go of the superior or ethnocentric attitude that keeps you separate from others—physically, mentally, emotionally, and spiritually. Become inclusive rather than exclusive. *We,* not *me.*

Look for opportunities to meet others who are on different life paths. Learn from them. Honor them. Just as you honor the path you chose, come to see that your path is one of many. Keep what feels right in your heart and dismiss that which is in discord with your internal self. Let your internal path guide your external path, not the other way around. Let your values and beliefs be honored in the path that you walk. Let your inner world be the compass that directs your outer world. Follow your heart.

In this way, your respect for all will contagiously inspire others to open their eyes and ears to the truth. In this way, you will fear none, and you will see external paths simply as paths either handed down from generation to generation or personally or internally created.

Create a healthy atmosphere in which you can flourish. This includes your own space, perhaps a room that reflects who you are at your deepest levels. This becomes an environment of mirrors (pictures, mementos, and objects of affection) constantly reminding you of what you deem important. What determines whether something is important is simply that it is important to you. It's your value judgment. Allow your environment to flow with your life.

Honor old traditions, if they are right for you. Create new traditions and stay in step with where you are on your life path. New traditions will give you a new vitality in your private, internal life. As you transcend in growth, fresh new traditions may become appropriate and valuable in solidifying your newfound level of consciousness. Dance to your own drum. In Ojibway, "all roads lead to the high place." We must respect all traditions, cultures, and religions—including our own.

Respect and admire the individuality of all of creation. Honor the awesome wonder that there are no two people, snowflakes, blades of grass, or anything in creation exactly alike. Hold freedom in highest regard, because our essence is a free spirit. If we stifle that, we slowly extinguish ourselves. Respect your right, my right, our right to create and follow the path that works best.

Keep your mind open wide. To feel better, we must think better, and to think better, we need to see life's opportunities, diversities, options, and choices clearly. Then life becomes a matter of not working harder, but living smarter. Life also becomes exciting as we become responsive and proactive, rather than insensitive and reactive.

Finally, learn to trust and love. Trust that your judgment is the best it can be at any moment, and love the joy of life, for soon we will be back home in Mother Earth's womb. If you do your best at every moment, you will have no regrets. There will be no need to beat yourself up for making a poor choice or decision, because you did your best. That is all any of us can do. We need to live in the present and set goals for the future. That's something we *can* do something about. The past is irreversible. What is, is!

Honor the paths of others, just as you now honor your path. Know what you can do and can't do. Give others the same trust that you give yourself. Love others, for that will never be cause for regret. Can you love too much? How so?

One World Family

We are one world family. A world family implies a great responsibility and commitment to one another. The pictures taken from outer space say more than words. There are no lines of demarcation on those pictures of Mother Earth. Rivers flow to oceans, which are blanketed with swirls of atmosphere. All is one. A family consists of two or more people who share goals and values, have long-term commitments to one another, and reside in the same dwelling place. A family is also a group that has a common heritage.

Ultimately, we are a family. As a world family, there is ultimately no distinction among us other than minor differences. Our characteristics are not differentiated by color, because we could line up every person in the world and the differences of color would blend one into the next. The Creator has no color, just warm energy light. We are of the same five-fingered species.

But there is more. As a world family, we share the same goals—to be loved and to love. We share the same values—to live, learn, and leave a legacy. We have a long-term commitment to each other, for we rely on one another for our health and happiness. We reside in the same dwelling place—planet Earth— and are interdependent. We breathe the same air and drink from the same waters. Our physical being is air and water; we are one within each other. We are linked, generation to generation.

We are one world family. I cannot exist without you. Despite denial and delusion, we are interrelated. We could trace our ancestries and find our paths all lead to one. We could go back to the beginning of time and find our common gene pool. We could acknowledge this connection. However, it is not necessary to even leave your home to see that you and I are related. Our food comes from the same earth. Open your refrigerator, and you will see the truth.

Someone grew, packaged, and shipped the apple you eat. Someone transported the meat. Someone engineered the refrigeration you now enjoy. Someone mined the materials to make your refrigerator. Someone built your home, which holds the refrigerator. Someone cut the trees to make the lumber for your home. Someone planted the trees. Someone provided you a job so you could purchase these things. The life you enjoy is the direct result of the work others did or provided for you. We are truly interdependent. I need you. You need me. It's *we*—not *me*.

As a world family, there are just so many of us. How can we possibly feel connected when it seems as though a sea of people, indistinguishable and separate, are all beyond our immediate life? To answer that, you need to look inside yourself for the truth. When you hear of a tragedy, are there moments (even a fleeting one) in which your heart goes out to the victims and their families? When you see jubilant fans on television, celebrating a victory for their country, does your heart celebrate alongside them, if only for a moment? When you wonder about your beginning and your end, do you not imagine the joining that will occur when you are finally near one another? Death is the ultimate life experience, for it joins us to the past, present, and future. All in one, one with all, generation to generation to generation.

We are all one world family. We are family.

Chapter Ten

Seven Generations

Watch the birds as they care for their young. Observe their focused attention, deliberate commitment, and discipline. The winged need to care, for care is needed. They listen to their needs and the needs of their young. It is a balanced listening. And the future is provided for.

We are at a turning point concerning our future generations. Look around you and notice. What do you see the younger generations needing? What do you see the older generations providing? Are we listening to the voices of today's young and tomorrow's elders?

The Iroquoian principle, that is held high for all to see and remember, attends to the needs of the seventh generation. Consider your actions and inactions in the light of the seventh generation. If they are helpful, then you would be wise to consider them. If they will be hurtful, then search for other alternatives. To fully grasp the extent of this wisdom, consider what the seventh generation would mean to you.

You are the first generation. Does your action (or inaction) help or hurt you? Your children are the second generation. Will your action (or inaction) help or hurt them? Your grandchildren are the third generation. Will your action (or inaction) help or hurt them? Your great-grandchildren are the fourth generation. Will your action (or inaction) help or hurt them? This is where most people's minds stop. After all, what we see of the future is what we are part of.

The seventh generation, however, takes you further along the space-time continuum. Consider that you will be present, just in a different form, to your great-great-grandchildren, who will be the fifth generation. Will your action (or inaction) help or hurt them? Your great-great-great-grandchildren will be the sixth generation. Will your action (or inaction) help or hurt them? Finally, your great-great-great-great-grandchildren will be the seventh generation.

With wisdom, consider all decisions in this light, and you will choose well. Always consider whether your action (or inaction) will help or hurt the seventh generation. Consider what tracks we will leave for our great-great-great-great-grandchildren. Will we have created better relationships and provided for these relationships in the best way possible? Or will we have hurt these relationships yet to be born and added to the cycle of abuse, exploitation, and self-centeredness?

At this very moment, you decide the legacy we will hand to our seventh generation. Every moment gives us opportunities to help or hurt. If you decide to give your child the necessary guidance in a loving way, have you helped or hurt your generation? Have you helped or hurt their generation? Now consider this action in the light of the future generations. Will your action likely be something to help or hurt? It is that simple. Matters small and matters large need the same deliberate attention shown above. If you are in a position of power or influence in any way, this teaching is especially vital. What will you do today that will help the seventh generation? What will you think about? Who will you become? How will you interact with those close to you? What will you change or keep the same? How will you make a difference? What will your legacy be?

To be a leader is to take responsibility for yourself, yet at the same time consider your actions in relation to others. As an inter-dependent partner, a leader is first concerned with how to help, not hurt. A leader considers all generations. With foresight and hindsight, a leader uses insight. A leader uses circular vision. He or she understands how the pebble in the water ripples out into ever-widening circles. Be of service, not a servant.

If starting tomorrow, all governments and leaders, including the United States Congress, would begin to make all their choices and decisions based on the seventh generation principle, what would change? *Everything* would change! Remember the seventh generation, and you will be a hero of many. Ignore the seventh generation, and you may be a part of its ruin.

Beyond Today

Time runs forward and backward. All part of the same con-tinuum, today is interrelated with what has been and what will be. Think beyond today in your decisions of great importance. See how your decisions were influenced by yesterday. See how you can influence tomorrow.

Our ancestors live in us today. What they did and did not do lives on in our daily lives. They all are part of our collective unconscious. Our ancestors are in perfect agreement and of one mind, because, now back in the spirit world, they know only pure truth. Our fathers, mothers, and ancestors walk our life path with us in our instincts and hearts. Together we are strong.

The past influences the present; nonetheless, we still exercise our free will. Although it is advisable to live in the present, unchecked satisfaction of your wants may not always be the best decision. We must think beyond today. Instant gratification, per-haps one of today's biggest problems, urges all of us to get what we can now. Manipulated by the advertising world, we seldom stop to consider what it is we actually need. And this is not limited to the unbridled consumption of physical things.

Our disposable society affects our relationships with others. Are others disposable, too? If we are not instantly gratified, are we not to move on to someone who will gratify our wants? Divorce rates skyrocket. Lasting and functional relationships are rare. Extended families are becoming a thing of the past. Concerned with today and how to get what we need and want, we have forgotten about investing in tomorrow. Foresight is clouded by indulgence.

Live today in the present, yet keep the consequences of your decisions in the forefront of your mind. With circular vision, see that foresight, hindsight, and insight will give you a global under-standing of how your choices influence today and tomorrow.

All that will be in the future is what we send ahead today. What are you sending ahead in your relationships? Where are you investing your time and effort? Are you depositing for the future? Or are you only withdrawing for the present? As always, it is a balancing act. Consider yourself to be part of the seven generations, but do not consider yourself to be *all* of the seven generations. Invest in yourself *and* invest in others.

Give your time and effort to those things that will ensure a healthy future. Do you know what you can give? Take a moment, right now, and think about various concepts that you believe will be valuable for the future. Write them down now. Now take one of these concepts (say, love, for example) and brainstorm ways in which you can help all seven generations. What can you do today that will promote love in the world? What can you do? Who will you offer love to? When? How?

Understand that today is already becoming yesterday. So plan for tomorrow, for your relationship with those yet to be born who depend on your decisions today. If we fail to plan, we plan to fail, and we will be as good as our plan.

Helpful, not Hurtful

All children understand the difference between something that is hurtful and something that is helpful. To make your decisions, you only need to ask the question "Is this helpful or hurtful?" Let *helpful, not hurtful* direct your every decision.

With such a basic language, we can come to understand the guiding principle of the seventh generation. Base all your decisions on this one question, and you will choose wisely. Too often, we don't ask, "Is this helpful or hurtful?" Instead, we ask, "Do I want it?" or "Can I afford it?" Change your indulgent questioning, and your results will change. Your future will change, too.

Please take this time to think of a decision that is weighing heavily on your mind. Perhaps it is an economic question, a family issue, a personal growth question, or a relationship question. Now take that question and consider your options. Consider the extent to which each option will be helpful or hurtful for all seven generations. Let this principle guide you into your decision-making process. Eventually, thinking this way will become more natural. Again, the more you practice, the more you become what you practice. Soon, you will easily and naturally think in terms of the seventh generation. Allow for risks; allow for opportunity costs. Consider all aspects of your dilemma. Let the helping principle guide you. Become less self-seeking and more far-reaching as you consider all seven generations. Help or hurt? That's the question.

Are You Having Fun Yet?

Just try to be angry, depressed, or worried while you sing freedom songs with a group. Just try to be angry, depressed, or worried while you play a board game with your family. Just try to be angry, depressed, or worried while you swing dance with your son or daughter. Just try to be angry, depressed, or worried while you participate in a musical. Just try. We dare you.

Impossible, isn't it? When we have fun, we can't be depressed or lonely. When we enjoy, we can't be angry. When we join with others in a creative effort, we can't be worried.

It seems impossible to harbor negative emotions when we honestly play, sing, dance, and create with others. We come into alignment when we purposefully seek activities that activate our minds, hearts, bodies, and spirits. Activities such as singing, dancing, and playing an instrument require all four aspects of our being. The more uplifting the song or game, the more likely we will shed the weights we carry around.

Have you ever been around someone who is so much fun, they simply light up the room? Bring that person to mind. What is it about them that creates such an atmosphere? Their fun is contagious, isn't it? Somehow, these people know how to seek and find the joy in life, the fun in life. A potentially boring meeting can become a hoot. A potentially difficult task can become a celebration of creative abilities.

Their ability to have fun helps all of us. What you need to do is exercise your fun-muscle. First of all, laugh. Seek things that you consider funny, a movie or a comic routine. Look for ways to have fun. Second, relax. Those who have fun are not uptight. They play. Watch a one- or two-year-old. They create play to have fun. Maybe they'll hide behind a blanket or hold their bare feet out for you to tickle. They take responsibility to create, participate, and engage others in fun. Too often, people are lazy when it comes to having fun. They want others to make fun for them. You must make your own fun!

Fun is a matter of perception. In every situation or circumstance, look for ways to perceive and experience that situation or circumstance without the seriousness. At the same time, find contradictions in life, which often are humorous. Make the substance of the situation secondary to enjoyment. Otherwise, the substance clouds the kernel of enjoyment hidden inside. Turn it inside out—in that process, substance becomes secondary and enjoyment becomes primary. For example: suppose you are sitting in a boring classroom and the professor demands a term paper, not to exceed one thousand words. So you submit to your professor a picture, because a picture is worth a thousand words. Now, in reality, this may not be such a wise idea. However to do this privately, mentally within yourself, or with a trusted friend would bring some fun, humor, and relief to you and the classroom. Hurray for internal dialogue.

Humor is nothing more than observing the contradictions in life and nurturing the ability to laugh. The more people you join, the greater the potential for fun. The more fun you have, the more contagious the fun is for others. Be careful, however, not to make others the target of your humor. What you find funny may be offensive to others.

Are you having fun yet? Are you enjoying life? Are you playing with your family? Do you sing? Do you dance? Are you laughing? Can you join a group with a common purpose to create something beautiful or inspiring? Fun is the essence and fragrance in life. Without fun, there is no sunshine.

What's more fun than fun? More fun!

Leaving a Legacy

Someday you will be someone's ancestor. You will leave a legacy. A legacy is what others remember you by, but it goes beyond your personality to the principles you uphold. What principles will survive your death? What truths do you stand by? What tracks will you leave for others to follow?

If you could sum up your reason for living in one sentence, what would it be? What is it that you really want to leave behind? Please take your time to answer this, as this may well be your legacy. Your legacy does not begin when the last shovel of dirt is tossed upon your grave. Your legacy begins now. Your legacy consists of all of the actions, values, and beliefs that you embrace today, all of which will remain after you are gone. What you do *does* matter. How will others remember you? What will continue after you are gone? What acts of love will you have contributed? How will the world be better because you were here? What has your carving knife of life whittled for future generations? How will it help? Will it hurt? What will you leave?

We all leave our tracks behind. What will be your tracks? Where will they lead others? What impression will you leave? What will be remembered? What will last? Will your presence last even after the sands of time erase your tracks? Think in terms of the end, for the end will then show you how to begin. If you look long and hard enough, you will uncover the tracks of your ancestors. They tell of long-lived truths; they are not for *me* but for *we*.

When the last breath escapes your body, what do you want to have left behind? A kinder, gentler world? A balanced, healthier world? Mended relationships? Healed relationships? Relationships of love? Relationships of meaning? What will be your relationship with relationships? Will you have discovered the sacred in all your relationships? Will you be distant or connected? Honoring and honorable? Will you respect all? Fear none? Will you still be present? Will you be attached or detached from future generations?

What kind of children, grandchildren, business, environment, government do you hope will survive your death? Realize that we all have influence. Although we cannot control people, we can influence people and policies. As history attests, we influence others by our example, not by what we say, but by what we do. Whom will you influence? Whom do you want to influence? What can you do to make and leave a positive influence?

Take this time to write down the important people in your life. Who are they? Where do they live? What would you like to say to them, if today were your last day? What principles do you wish to communicate to them? What example are you leaving them to notice and wonder about? What communication have you promoted that lets each of you see the other more clearly? What love do you wish to express? Have you given your presence?

The greatest gift we have to give another is our presence. Maybe that's why our pets are so important to us. They constantly give us this gift. We get to know only those with whom we spend time. With whom do you need to invest more time and energy? Who needs your comforting presence? What do you need to tell them?

What is your epitaph?

Your relationships are indeed sacred. You are sacred. May these words accelerate your journey into loving yourself and others more completely, loving the universe and your God completely. The seventh generation silently awaits your momentary decisions.

What will you do today to heal the world? Every moment is a gift. You are both the receiver of breath and giver of your attention. What will you give from your life today to heal the world? What will you receive in your life today to help heal the world?

Remember the ripples. Each momentary decision, everything you do or don't do matters. You matter. We matter. The seventh generation matters. Reach into and beyond self in order to experience the joy of living. You are the creator of your life. You hold the pebble in your hand.

Bibliography / Recommended Reading

Campbell, Joseph. *The Hero With a Thousand Faces.* Princeton, NJ: Princeton University Press, 1949.

Chopra, Deepak. *The Path to Love.* New York: Harmony Books, 1997.

Covey, Stephen R. *The 7 Habits of Highly Effective People.* New York: Simon and Schuster, 1989.

The Dalai Lama. *Ethics for the New Millennium.* New York: Riverhead Books, 1999.

Davies, Paul. *About Time: Einstein's Unfinished Revolution.* New York: Simon and Schuster, 1995.

Doss, Ram. *Still Here: Embracing Aging, Changing, and Dying.* New York: Riverhead Books, 2001.

Dyer, Wayne W. *Your Sacred Self.* New York: HarperCollins Publishers, 1995.

Frankl, Viktor E. *Man's Search for Meaning: An Introduction to Logotherapy.* Boston: Beacon Press Books, 1959.

Galbraith, John Kenneth. *The Affluent Society,* 3rd ed. Boston: Houghton Mifflin Company, 1976.

Hanh, Thich Nhat. *The Wisdom of Thich Nhat Hanh.* Boston: Beacon Press and Parallax Press, 2000.

Jones, Blackwolf and Gina. *Listen to the Drum.* Center City, MN: Hazelden Publishing, 1995.

Jones, Blackwolf and Gina. *Earth Dance Drum.* Center City, MN: Hazelden Publishing, 1996.

Jones, Gina, Maryellen Baker, and Mildred Schuman. *The Healing Blanket.* Center City, MN: Hazelden Publishing, 1998.

Lee, Sally. *The Throwaway Society.* New York: An Impact Book, 1990.

MacEachern, Diane. *Save Our Planet: 750 Everyday Ways You Can Help Clean Up the Earth.* New York: Dell Publishing, 1990.

Mother Teresa. *In My Own Words.* Liguori, MO: Liguori Publications, 1996.

Rivers, Frank. *The Way of the Owl: Succeeding With Integrity in a Conflicted World.* San Francisco: HarperCollins Publishers, 1996.

Satir, Virginia. *Conjoint Family Therapy.* Palo Alto, CA: Science and Behavior Books, 1983.

Satir, Virginia. *Self Esteem.* Millbrae, CA: Celestial Arts, 1970.

Schwartz, Morrie. *Letting Go.* New York: Dell Publishing, 1996.

About the Authors

Blackwolf and Gina Jones are presenters and teachers of age-old wisdom. Blackwolf Jones is an elder of Ojibway heritage and, as a licensed psychotherapist, blends ancient tribal healing remedies with contemporary approaches. He is an international speaker who brings an electrifying and charismatic presence to workshops and seminars. Gina, of Mohawk and European ancestry, is a middle-school teacher, who also writes fiction (*The Healing Blanket*). Gina presents at various gatherings and actively practices the creative arts. Authors of *Listen to the Drum, The Healing Drum,* and *Earth Dance Drum,* Blackwolf and Gina Jones bring years of experience and training to recovery through Native American spirituality and life principles.